On leaving school, Jon Sandifer travelled for six years through 52 countries – mostly by land and sea. It was during this journey that he became interested in Eastern philosophy and healing and, on his return to Britain, he trained in oriental diagnosis, macrobiotics and Shiatsu with Japanese master Michio Kushi. In 1983 he was appointed Director of the Kushi Institute in London and in 1988 became one of Kushi's 'Senior Teachers', a title held by only 15 people in the world.

Also by Jon Sandifer

Acupressure for Health, Vitality and First Aid
Feng Shui Astrology

THE
10
DAY
RE-BALANCE
PROGRAMME

A Unique New Life Plan to Dramatically Improve Your Health and Inner Well-Being

JON SANDIFER

RIDER
London · Sydney · Auckland · Johannesburg

1 3 5 7 9 10 8 6 4 2

First published in 1998 in Great Britain by Rider,
an imprint of Ebury Press, Random House,
20 Vauxhall Bridge Road, London SW1V 2SA

Random House Australia (Pty) Limited
20 Alfred Street, Milsons Point, Sydney,
New South Wales 2061, Australia

Random House New Zealand Limited
18 Poland Road, Glenfield,
Auckland 10, New Zealand

Random House South Africa (Pty) Limited
Endulini, 5A Jubilee Road, Parktown 2193, South Africa

Random House UK Limited Reg. No. 954009

Papers used by Rider Books are natural, recyclable
products made from wood grown in sustainable forests.

Typeset by SX Composing DTP, Rayleigh, Essex
Printed by CPD, Wales

A CIP catalogue record for this book
is available from the British Library

ISBN 0-7126-7136-6

For my parents
Mim and Sandy

ACKNOWLEDGEMENTS

My heartfelt thanks to Michio and Aveline Kushi whose books and seminars individually inspired me to experience life from a yin/yang perspective.

For Bill Tara, founder of the East West Centre in London, for his teaching, support and constant challenge of my understanding of the paradoxical qualities of yin and yang.

For Shizuko Yamamoto for sharing her unique knowledge of Shiatsu which has benefitted me enormously these past twenty years.

For Brian Roet and Matthew Manning for introducing me to other perspectives on self-healing that I value and integrate into my life.

For one of my oldest friends, John Cairns, with whom I shared many adventures in our youth, for introducing me to Rider Books

For my editor, Judith Kendra, who saw the potential for this book and has encouraged me throughout the whole process.

For my sister Mary, for her courageous gift to me of one of her kidneys in 1995, enabling me to return to full health. No words can express my gratitude.

For my wife Renata for her unconditional love, support and patience these past few years.

I thank you all, and also my friends, colleagues, students and clients who have contributed to my knowledge by sharing their own unique experiences.

CONTENTS

Part One: The Dynamics of Balance

1 What is Change?   3

2 Yin and Yang – The Navigation Tools   21

3 Understanding Ourselves   32

4 Oriental Diagnosis: Self-Assessment   65

Part Two: The Programme

5 Making Changes   87

6 Step One: Knowing Who and Where You Are   98

7 Step Two: Planning the Voyage   124

8 Step Three: Setting Off   142

9 Where to Go from Here   227

  Resources/Food Glossary   232

PART ONE

The Dynamics of Balance

1

What is Change?

'There are risks and costs to a programme of action. But they are far less than the long range risks and cost of comfortable in-action.'

J. F. Kennedy

There are times in all of our lives when we can feel stuck in a rut. Common symptoms that are a sign of stagnation include boredom and tiredness. When we feel uninspired it is natural for us to need a new freshness and a polarity with what we are doing. When we feel exhausted, overwhelmed and stressed, we need time and space to take stock of the situation, to recreate our health, our creativity and our dream. Frequently, we only really notice that we require change when our back is to the wall – manifesting as 'I can't cope', 'I want to change my job', 'I need to be out of this relationship' or 'I need to move house'.

The longer we delay making changes the more chronic our condition becomes and we can begin to believe that this is all our life is about. On the other hand, if we were able to see this phase of our life relative to our past, present and future, then we would be able to perceive that what we are really experiencing is a turning point – the potential for change.

The key to success in this 10-day re-balancing programme is the recovery of our intuition. We are all born with this inherent skill and throughout our lives its quality is dependent on our current health. Whether we are feeling too busy and stressed out or are tired and despondent – our general condition and health pervades our intuition and we frequently make decisions that further emphasize the imbalance. Using the information in this book, which has been drawn from many aspects of oriental healing and wisdom, you will be able to create the opportunity during one 10-day period to re-discover and strengthen your intuition. Like a good New Year's resolution, we intuitively know what we need to do to bring us back on track but frequently fail due to outside pressure and distractions. During this ten days you have the opportunity to create an oasis in the busyness of your life which will allow you to really listen to what you need and undertake the practical steps to bring about beneficial change.

WHY THIS PROGRAMME IS UNIQUE

Our physiology as human beings is primarily the same as that of our ancestors 5,000-10,000 years ago. However, the challenges that we now face are different. For example, our nervous systems are facing increasing burdens due to our high-tec, fast moving, pressurized lifestyle. But while these may be under increased strain today, our circulatory systems are not challenged in the same way that they were for our forebears. We use public transport and cars to go about our business and rarely face the challenges of the elements any longer. Our offices, homes, shopping precincts and even our vehicles are heated. Where our ancestors' nervous systems were challenged by hunting, warfare or the vagaries of the weather, ours face a seemingly constant deluge of information and speedy demands.

Yet, in spite of this change, the principles of discovering health, harmony and balance outlined in traditional oriental texts are of as much value today as they were when they were first conceived thousands of years ago and later written down. By getting to grips with the principles of these systems and applying them to our modern lifestyles, we can still achieve the potential for breaking the stagnation in our lives that could already be creating or manifesting as dis-ease.

A unique facet of this book is that it will enable you to gain a fresh insight into your current position, a clear view of what you would like to achieve and a choice of practical guidelines to fulfil your new dream or direction. You will also be undertaking this work by yourself, without the intervention of a health practitioner.

Changes that are hasty, extreme, reactionary or badly thought out, inevitably have no lasting effect. Often the more extreme we are the quicker we pull out of a programme of change and revert to our old patterns with more intensity than before. There has to be a point between the one extremity of making violent or reactionary change and the other of hopeless indifference to any form of change.

Most cultures and traditional religions in our world have incorporated into their practice some form of self-reflection that is applied over an extended period every year, Lent or Ramadan for example.

This is because it is hard to take stock of a situation in the heat of action – far easier if we can create an oasis of time to reflect and chart our course. Part of the purpose of this programme is to simplify and examine areas of our lives that we wish to change – and ten days is not too great a demand. The intention is not to 'get a result' at the end of the ten days but to regain our intuition so that our future actions are born out of a fresh, new perspective.

Biologically there is sense in this argument also. We draw our fundamental nutrition from food, liquid and oxygen – without these we cannot survive. By making fundamental changes in these three areas over a ten-day period we can begin to bring about change on a cellular level, starting with our blood. In terms of volume almost half of our blood is made up of plasma and this renews itself approximately every ten days. Our blood in turn is nourishing our organs, our nervous system, recharging, rebuilding and revitalizing every moment of the day. As our blood is refreshed and our organs begin to benefit from this new change (the heart, the lungs, the kidneys, etc.) it is inevitable that this new-found vitality will permeate our nervous system and therefore our awareness, what we might call our consciousness. In other words, ten days is a minimum period to clear the decks, sweep away the cobwebs and see clearly where you are and what you want to take on.

GUIDELINES FOR CHANGE

As human beings, our ability to 'respond' has a great deal to do with the state of our nervous system. In the Orient the nervous system is seen as a physicalized form of our central, spiritual channel, and this channel is regarded as an antenna for picking up the natural charge we receive from our immediate environment. We constantly receive information and make decisions and judgements based on what we perceive. When we are tired, stressed, intoxicated, we do not perceive the world clearly and our actions can reflect that. So there really is a biological basis in the health of our nervous system. Part of the work that we will cover in this book is intended to sharpen and clarify the nervous system during a ten-day period to enable you to see clearly what is going on around you and base your future dreams and judgement on that.

Sometimes it can be all too easy to blame outside factors as to why we feel stuck or incapable of change. We can blame our job, our home life, our dwelling space, our relationships, pressures from family responsibilities and even old patterns in our life for causing our current impasse. Undoubtedly, many of these factors play a part in our outlook on the world, and we shall see later in this book how we can break some of these patterns and thereby create new openings and opportunities for change in all areas of our lives.

Problems, difficulties and challenges can be our greatest teachers. Although seemingly unpleasant at the time there is undoubtedly a learning process within the trauma. I have personally found that when we sideline or avoid the challenge it will inevitably recur – often with greater ferocity or in a different shape or form. Until we really grasp the nettle of the problem it will continue to linger and subtly drain us until it is resolved.

Ultimately, what we need to remember is that our bodies and our environment are excellent self-balancing systems. Basically, our body is on our side. It does not intend to be an enemy or get in the way of our progress. Given appropriate fuel and exercise it will find its own state of balance without undue tinkering. The same is largely true of our environment. It is a self-balancing, self-regenerating system that the more it is adjusted will ultimately cause imbalances elsewhere within the eco-system. Getting in touch with this 'cellular' memory is part of the purpose of this programme.

A BRIEF AUTOBIOGRAPHY

Born in 1953 I was raised on the coast of Kenya, enjoying a wonderful childhood in this tropical paradise. From a young age I enjoyed the open spaces, the opportunity to explore, big wide open skies and plenty of sunshine! Later, I went to a British public school for eight years and, when I was seventeen, embarked on an expedition with four friends to the island of Spitzbergen in the Arctic Circle. It was an awesome experience to live for six weeks isolated and unsupported, miles from civilization. At times the experience was purely spiritual, at others it was a hard, physical slog, and sometimes it seemed as if we were on the set of *Lord of the Flies*! On my return to England and to school I found that I could not reintegrate. The experience had left me hungry for new horizons, new experiences and a desire to find out more about the world than could be taught at school. Within twenty-four hours I had 'borrowed' my basic survival equipment from the expedition, several kilos of dehydrated food and, without a word to anyone, I hitchhiked to Dover, took a ferry to France and began what was to become a six-year adventure – travelling around the world by my wits and on a limited budget.

Pretty soon I discovered that it wasn't how much money I had in my pocket or how much food in my belly but my attitude and outlook that helped me discover positive experiences. If when I was soaked, hungry and cold I allowed an air of despondency to creep in then I only seemed to attract more negative experiences. If on the other hand, I looked on the bright side, I could find uplifting signs all around. In times of difficulty I used to sing a song I heard on the radio years ago:

I have four wheels on my wagon and I'm still rolling along,
The Cherokees are chasing me but I'm singing a happy song.

The lyric continues to have three wheels, then two wheels and finally only one wheel on your wagon. When I had my back against the wall I would always sing the first line, and never allow myself to go with less than four wheels on my wagon!

When I was eighteen years old, a fellow traveller lent me a copy of Lao Tzu's *Tao Te Ching* – a Chinese classic which forms the basis of Taoism. The inference is that we live in a changing world and that all phenomena are interconnected. I would obtain hours of pleasure from reading and re-reading the same verse, often gaining a new insight when I returned to it several months later.

In 1977, while working in Germany, I had a recurrence of a childhood ear problem. Specialists in Germany diagnosed cholesteatoma and recommended that I had immediate surgery. I returned to London and, with the help of my father who is a doctor, received rapid and expert help. However, the outcome of the operation was not successful and, warned that the problem would soon recur, I began to investigate alternatives. I had read some literature by George Ohsawa and Michio Kushi on the subject of macrobiotics and decided that the holistic view that they presented was more my cup of tea.

However, my initial consultation with a macrobiotic expert

gave me little inspiration. He said that the problem was with my kidneys and that I should apply a ginger compress to them, eat plenty of brown rice and aduki beans. At this point, losing interest, my gaze fell on his bookshelf to see what he read. It was there that I spotted a copy of the *Tao Te Ching* and, to my delight, when I asked him if he had read the book, discovered that it was the basis of his whole philosophy. In that moment I felt I was 'home and dry'.

From then on, I studied macrobiotic cooking, oriental diagnosis, Shiatsu massage, yin yang philosophy and, within three years, I was a teacher and later a macrobiotic counsellor and Shiatsu practitioner. To the amazement of the ear specialist, within eight months the symptoms had disappeared. Over the next few years I continued to teach and practise what is essentially an oriental folk remedy system with an all-embracing philosophy of the connection between mind, body and spirit.

A new and more interesting challenge faced me in 1988 when I was diagnosed as having adult heredity polycystic kidney disease – a genetic disorder that manifests in slow kidney failure needing the eventual use of a dialysis or a possible transplant. The diagnosis and the prognosis challenged all that I believed or thought I knew. Apart from the ear problem I had never visited a doctor and was convinced that I knew all the answers. By 1993 it became clear that I needed dialysis and this was a turning point in my education and my life as I began to blend the best of both alternative and conventional medicine. My sister Mary, to whom I am eternally indebted, offered me one of her kidneys, and in 1995 I had a successful kidney transplant that enables me now to live a normal life. I still face a lifetime working with orthodox medicine and heavy duty anti-rejection drugs, but using the principles that will be outlined in the next few chapters I have been able to successfully balance my health so far.

THE MARGINS

A column on the left-hand side of a page where you can scribble 'what if', 'must study further' or 'research this later', a margin is partially intended for our own discoveries, thoughts and questions. In many books the text comprises two main areas: what we already know and material of which we have no knowledge but could gain access if we chose to study further. The 'margin' could represent 'what you don't even know you do not know'. It represents, therefore, new ideas, new distinctions, new research, and areas of life that we are not aware of at the moment. In this book, I invite you to join me in the 'margins' and, even, to extend them. Furthermore, I suggest you imagine you know very little about the body or human health.

When I first studied with Mr Kushi he emphasized that any information presented needed to be discussed, questioned and debated amongst students and teachers alike and I agree with him in this. It is this capacity for re-search and continual questioning – coming from the Zen concept of a beginners' mind to all questions and challenges – that forms the basis of oriental philosophy. I offer you a similar invitation. While reading this book, push open the margins and see what you can discover that is perhaps fresh and new. Try not to make the information sit necessarily with your concept of health, the body or spirit. This is not to say that what I present is the only approach, or even a unique approach, but it is another angle from which we can understand ourselves and our current condition.

WHAT IS HEALTH?

Posing this question in a seminar or a consultation inevitably brings a variety of responses. They include 'an absence of symptoms', 'an absence of disease', 'a state of mind', 'adaptability', etc. The definition of health that inspired me twenty years ago was entitled by George Ohsawa the 'seven levels of health'.

Ohsawa himself wrote some three hundred books in Japanese and twenty in French over a forty-year period, while introducing the oriental model of health to Westerners. In the 1930s while living in France he began to teach meditation, oriental philosophy, oriental medicine, macrobiotic cooking and continued to inspire his students to take responsibility for their own well-being. Here, I have drawn from his definitions but used my own interpretation.

1 No tiredness/fatigue

I would estimate that over 50 per cent of clients that I have met regard tiredness and fatigue as the major reasons they are looking for changes in their life. Essentially, these are symptoms of our modern lifestyle which while exciting, challenging and satisfying on one level can leave us drained and exhausted. There are two types of fatigue – the acute and the chronic. Acute fatigue is fundamentally the kind of tiredness we deserve when we have been working and exercising hard, receiving plenty of fresh air, or, on the other hand, when we have overeaten, sat in a stuffy room all day or had a poor night's sleep. This kind of tiredness can easily be resolved by simple eating and one or two nights' good sleep. There is something almost satisfying about the acute form of tiredness when we have taken a long exhilarating walk in the country and fall asleep almost as soon as our head hits the pillow.

It is the second form of fatigue, the chronic, that is far more insidious. It develops slowly and we begin to think that it is normal. The chronic fatigue begins to permeate all areas of our life and creativity. We may be working on a new project but find it difficult to feel inspired because we lack the freshness and vitality that it requires. Our enthusiasm to socialize and take risks begins to minimalize. I call this state of being the 'duvet' syndrome, when our world or universe seems to end at the edges of our bed. Rather than taking an outward look at the world we acquire a more introspective view, enjoying our sleep, our solitude and our space. Hopefully, this is a temporary phase while we recoup and regain our strength. If we indulge in the duvet syndrome for too long we cease to take any interest in what is going on beyond our home, beyond our street, beyond our culture and this leads us into inevitable isolation and despondency.

Imagine when you are tired how your energy will affect your enthusiasm for simple functions like cooking. It is essential that our spark gets into the cooking process! This means that when we are tired our cooking is tired and we frequently end up creating a 'tired' meal. This doesn't further improve our condition as we are creating much more of the same. Not having the energy to cook a hot, vitalizing meal in the evening will inevitably lead us to having something that is either quick or cold and soggy to prepare – thus perpetrating and continuing a spiral of fatigue. Another area of our life that tiredness can effect is sex. Admittedly sex is not high on our list of survival priorities like breathing, drinking, eating and sleeping; but our capacity and energy for sex is very much symptomatic of our current well-being. There are many environmental factors that can cause us unnecessary fatigue, including overheated homes and offices, lack of fresh air where we sleep, excessive amounts of electricity in our homes, too much time spent on computer systems, certain types of lighting and environmental distractions such as noise, traffic and pollution. Many of these factors we can choose to label the cause of our fatigue, but a healthy person will attempt to adapt to these challenges or make fundamental changes within their environment or lifestyle in order to compensate.

I believe that the mind plays a large role in our creation of fatigue. When you suggest to someone that they need a little more exercise their response is that it will make them more tired. I remember on one occasion telephoning a colleague to invite him for a meal on Friday evening, his response was that it was now Tuesday and that he would inevitably be tired by Friday and would like already to schedule another evening! This kind of tiredness, as well as visualizing its occurrence, can really limit our potential for health and happiness.

If we are living in a four seasons climate then in many ways it is wise to observe and to a certain degree imitate other four seasons mammals. If you are lucky enough to be flexible in your employment schedule it is easier to put in longer hours in the spring and summer and wiser to cut back your hours in the late autumn and winter to conserve your energy during the more dormant months. The industrialized world does not take this into account and we are all expected to work at least forty hours per week whether it is high summer or mid-winter. However, traditional farmers would have put in perhaps sixteen hours a day in the summer and had more time indoors and less working in the winter. This all helps to conserve our energy, refresh us and revitalize our health.

2 Good appetite

Appetite in this context of defining health goes beyond our interest in food. It includes all ares of our life that require daily involvement. Our potential for expressing ourselves creatively has a great deal to do with appetite – our interest and our hunger to develop new ideas. Appetite plays a part in our relationships, in our sex life, in our social life. Perhaps another word for appetite is curiosity. The people in our society who have the greatest appetite and the greatest curiosity are undoubtedly children. They are always on the move discovering new facets of the world, exploring their space and constantly enquiring 'why?' You only have to spend a day or two with a healthy three year old to get a clear definition of appetite – whether it is their constant demands for food and drink or their enquiries into why this and why that? In our early years this curiosity and appetite can be encouraged, while equally it can be discouraged. When a three year old constantly asks the question 'why?' a parent has the choice of patiently explaining or responding impatiently – 'ask the other parent' or 'wait until you go to school'. It is possible that this appetite is dampened at an early age by a parent who does not take their child's curiosity seriously or does not encourage them to find out more.

Some of the youngest and most flexible adults that I have met have enormous curiosity and appetite for life. We all know elderly friends and relatives who in their retirement take up a new project or learn to use the computer or begin communicating with others through the Internet. On the other hand, there are adults far younger who have shut down their curiosity to new avenues as they embark on their safe career, guaranteed income, mortgage repayments, etc. They are often like a train on a railway track going in one particular direction with no opportunity to make a detour or stop. They have completed their education and there is little encouragement to research or develop beyond that point. A good appetite and a curiosity for life is very much like the oriental model of Zen mind – the beginner's mind. The capacity to take all events and situations at face value, to see them with fresh eyes and to exercise one's judgement from the moment rather than from past experience or learning.

3 Good sleep

Undoubtedly, when we are tired, stressed and under pressure it will effect our sleep pattern. Sleep plays an important part in overall health, helping us to recharge and revitalize our nervous system and ourselves. There is no set rule or requirement as to how much we need; it is a very individual requirement. If we are living in a four seasons climate then it is wise to increase the amount of sleep in the autumn and winter months and decrease the amount in the spring and summer. Catching up with sleep at weekends or even having a siesta can be equally beneficial. It is a lot easier in the summer to party until very late, take a few hours sleep and still get to work feeling reasonably refreshed. Try and do this deep in the winter and you will inevitably feel tired for several days. Biologically, we seem to be very linked to the seasons and the climatic conditions and need to adjust our sleep patterns accordingly.

Good sleep also relates to the quality of the sleep that we enjoy. A symptom of good health is when we can fall asleep within a few minutes of our head touching the pillow. Tossing and turning for hours is not a good sign. Dreaming or not dreaming is not significant, but nightmares and sleep disturbances are signs that we are under excessive stress. A healthy definition of sleep is not however many hours we have but that it is adequate, that we fall asleep fairly quickly, that we are undisturbed by nightmares and visits to the toilet and that we awake refreshed without the need of an alarm clock.

4 Good memory

This level of health can be divided into three parts. To begin with there is what I call mechanical memory. This is our ability to remember dates, appointments, telephone numbers and our daily commitments without necessarily having to rely on memory joggers. When we are in good health our mechanical memory is very sharp and we rarely forget appointments or important pieces of information. If, on the other hand, we are not feeling on top form then we can appear to ourselves and to others 'scatty'. It is easy to forget where we have left an important item; we may forget an appointment or fail to fulfil an earlier commitment. When these symptoms and signs start to occur it is wise to take stock of our current state of well-being and see how we can make changes.

The second quality of memory I call biological memory. Without any doubt, our body has the remarkable capacity for balancing itself without any conscious effort from ourself. Biological memory is connected with the deep-seated memory that is within every cell and structure in our body. Are you constantly reminding yourself to breathe? Do you need to remind your heart to beat? If you go out this evening and drink one and a half bottles of wine, follow this up with a couple of brandies, take a cheap meal home to consume in front of the television at 1 o'clock in the morning, you are undoubtedly putting your whole system under strain. However, when you go to bed in whatever state you find yourself, your body is going to make an all-out effort without any intervention from you to re-balance the situation. Your digestive system will be awake all night; your liver and kidneys will work hard on regaining a balance within your blood; and undoubtedly if you put this level of strain on your system you are going to feel tired the morning after these major systems worked on overtime. Whatever challenges you throw at yourself it is important to remember that your unique self-balancing system is dedicated to your survival. It is only when this system is constantly challenged that more chronic or degenerative dis-ease can set in. I believe that most chronic illness could be defined as 'cellular amnesia', indicating that our body has or is experiencing a temporary loss of memory. Regaining this biological memory has a profound effect on our health and well-being. The secret lies in knowing our capacity and fuelling and challenging ourselves in a way that is appropriate to our make-up.

The third kind of memory I define as spiritual memory – knowing who you are, where you are and being totally at ease with your current situation. We all experience this from time to time. Spiritual memory manifests when we have no fear or worry in the present and feel that we are on course to a successful happy future. It can also manifest as a feeling of being at one with the current situation, that everything occurring in your life is perfect and on target. I used to experience the feeling as a child after a particularly exciting day out, after winning a prize at school or having completed a project that was satisfying and challenging. Equally, we have that feeling when we watch a beautiful sunset, fall in love or see our team win! This feeling of security and lack of fear for the future is my definition of spiritual memory.

5 Good humour

A healthy manifestation of this level is flexibility: our ability to adapt to new situations, new challenges and to the obstacles that may appear in life. For some it is the ability to see the funny side of life's challenges and being able to cope with change. When we are tired, run down or stuck we can lose our flexibility and become increasingly irritable. Being irritable, impatient and losing our temper at the slightest inconvenience are sure signs of being under stress. This is not to say that anger is a 'bad' emotion. Anger can be very powerful when we direct it creatively; for example, we can harness individual or collective anger in demonstrating a particular belief. Anger used as an initiating emotion can be a very powerful vehicle for change. However, being intolerant, angry and irritable on a regular basis can lead to a deeper more draining and more insidious state which I define as resentment.

Resentment can be an enormous drain on our creative capacity and on our general well-being. It is the symptom of an unresolved issue in our life. It takes enormous energy from us to retain the resentment, energy that could be used more creatively in health and well-being. Letting go of resentment, developing a spirit of forgiveness and tolerance, are the first steps toward dissolving the physically and emotionally exhausting qualities that resentment can bring. There is a parallel between what it costs to maintain resentment and that of a leak in the fuel pipe on your car. It is draining and costing you all the time. In Chapter 8 we shall be looking at a visualization exercise aimed at clearing resentment should it exist.

6 Precision in thought and action

All our thoughts, actions and responses to our environment need to involve our nervous system. This system acts as an antenna for picking up stimuli from our environment, interpreting the signals and initiating and completing action. When our nervous system is tired or dulled then our response is equally low-key. Poor reception will undoubtedly result in poor action and inevitably costs us in terms of mistakes. Keeping our nervous system sharp and alert really helps us to ascertain clearly where we are and where we are going. Having a variety of different activities in our daily routine helps to train this system – plenty of mental activity coupled with challenges that are more physical. A combination of the two in the form of, say, practising a martial art, is excellent training for the nervous system.

In today's world we blame much of our unhappiness on stress. Why is it then that some friends seem to thrive in pressurized situations and others seem to fall apart? When any system is weak or overloaded it will only take a little more pressure for it to become 'stressed' and begin to break down. The continued incidence in the Western world of so-called 'road rage' is symptomatic of a breakdown of this level of health. Some drivers, under enormous pressures at work, time constraints and other responsibilities, find that the challenges of modern-day driving are the last straw. Seemingly small incidents turn into major excuses to release their stress, their anger or their frustration.

7 Gratitude

Ohsawa saw this as the most challenging level of health and believed that its opposite manifestation, of arrogance, could be the most detrimental. Gratitude, here, is being fully responsible for our lives, our health, our current situation. Being grateful for challenges and difficulties helps to remove any tendency to blame something or someone else for our situation. Having a sense of gratitude for the learning experiences that challenges can provide undoubtedly helps to dissolve any sense that we are powerless. If we are going to initiate some kind of change within our life we need to be clear from the beginning that this is our responsibility and that whatever has stimulated us to make changes is essentially our teacher and in many ways an inspiration. For this we can, to some measure, be grateful.

Summary

What I have learnt to appreciate from this definition of health is that the first four levels (fatigue, appetite, sleep and memory) are closely linked to how we are currently living and are relatively easy to change. However, if the symptoms are left unattended, the more chronic patterns begin to set in and re-balancing becomes a bigger challenge as our condition changes from acute to chronic. However, we cannot change our attitude, our sense of humour or the state of our nervous system effectively without making fundamental changes to our basic health – vitality, appetite, sleep and memory. Regaining our vitality and curiosity are essential first steps in the re-balancing programme, paving the way to benefit from our refreshed intuition.

NAVIGATION

Setting out on any programme of change can be like any other journey we undertake. There is a parallel here between initiating change and setting sail across the sea. The 'compass' that I will present for the navigation exercise in this book are the oriental concepts of yin and yang. Their qualities and the various expressions of these principals will be outlined in Chapter 2. Essentially they can provide us with a very dynamic view of ourselves, our situation and our intended journey.

The first thing to consider when contemplating a sea voyage is the kind of vessel you will undertake the journey in. I shall call this our constitution and in Chapter 3 will explain how to assess this using oriental diagnosis. Then before setting sail, we need to check on the condition of the vessel, the state of its machinery, ropes, supplies and fastenings. The difference between constitution and condition is that the constitution relates to the structure, capacity and potential based on how the vessel was constructed. For example, there is a constitutional difference between a schooner and a plywood sailing dingy. Would you undertake to cross the Atlantic ocean in November in a plywood dingy? Knowing our constitution and its condition helps us to determine what kind of journey or direction would be wise.

When contemplating a journey it is important to discover first exactly 'where' you are. In Chapter 6 you will be able to chart clearly your current state of well-being through various processes of self-reflection and self-diagnosis.

Sailors and navigators do not set out into the ocean without their destination or goal in mind. The results of any change of course or change of direction in our life needs to be coupled with a clear sense of what you want to achieve. The exercises in Chapter 7 are designed to help us visualize a future into which we intend to live.

The next task is to plot a course from 'a' to 'b' and there are infinite ways in which you could make the journey. By knowing your capacity, your condition, your current position and your intended destination, it is far easier to decide which course of action you wish to take in order to achieve your goal. Chapter 8 outlines the various options which we can use and correlates them to our current condition. It is very like a chart on board a ship. You can see in pencil the intended route that the skipper meant to take but there are other pencil lines which indicate the variables a navigator needs to take into account. These include the direction and strength of the wind, the state of the tide, and the strength and direction of any currents. All these factors, together with any errors of judgement and navigation, lead to inevitable deviations from the straight line from 'a' to 'b'. Chapter 9 deals with the ups and downs that can occur when we initiate change, the kinds of distractions that can push us off course, and how to evaluate in future situations where we are and what systems can we employ again should we wish to make another journey.

2

Yin and Yang –
The Navigation Tools

The concept of yin and yang can provide fascinating insights into 'who' and 'where' we are regarding our health and current direction in life. Yin and yang can provide us with a dynamic set of principles which can be as applicable today as they were in the early civilizations of China and Tibet. Today the connotations of yin and yang are associated with acupuncture, Feng Shui, Taoism and oriental esoteric teachings, and their principles are just as valid as they were thousands of years ago. In this chapter we can take a look at how they operate and how practical they are as tools to understand the dynamics of change.

Yin and yang are simply terms to describe opposite qualities of phenomena in our environment. The traditional peoples of the world understood that they lived in a changing environment and used them to reflect this fact. We still live, work and operate in such a world – only the changes occur faster, under more pressure and with more far-reaching results.

One of the best examples of the unconscious yin and yang in our lives is when, as very young children, we began to distinguish and identify the world around us. As newborn babies we perceive our immediate environment using essentially what we could now call yin/yang distinctions. For example, we become aware of sensations that are hot or cold. We make our mothers aware when we are either hungry or full. We notice when we are wet and dry and can perceive the difference between light and dark and an environment that is quiet or noisy. As we grow and develop we begin to develop opinions based on what we like or dislike. This can include a preference for sweet rather than salty foods, hard rather than soft-textured foods. As we begin to communicate with words we can communicate our own opinions regarding people that we like or dislike, books that we wish to read, clothes that we wish to wear and others that we do not. All these youthful distinctions are parallel to early civilization's view of the environment in which they lived.

The dynamic application of the principles of yin and yang form the basis of traditional oriental philosophy and its application in all areas of life. The concept itself can probably be traced back to the influence of three seminal books written thousands of years ago in China. The first was the classic of divination called the *I Ching* which does not mention yin and yang as such, but points out that humanity exists between heaven (yang) and earth (yin) and is influenced by the forces of both. The underlying principle is the concept of change, that life flows like a river without any pause regardless of night or day.

Another source in the development of the concept of yin and yang is undoubtedly the work of Lao Tzu and his treatise known as the *Tao Te Ching*. Like the *I Ching*, the *Tao Te Ching* does not present yin and yang per se, but alludes to the qualities of opposites in nature and their role in creating all phenomena. In the second verse of his classic, Lao Tzu writes, 'The hidden and the obvious give birth to each other.' 'Difficult and easy complement each other.' 'Long and short exhibit each other.' 'High and low set measure to each other.' 'Voice and sound harmonize each other.' 'Back and front follow each other.' In verse 11 he again touches on the yin/yang concept in his expression that 'thirty spokes converge upon a single hub; it is on the hole in the centre that the use of the cart hinges . . . We make a vessel from a lump of clay; it is the empty space within the vessel that makes itself useful . . . We make doors and windows for a room; but it is these empty spaces that make the room liveable. Thus, while the tangible has advantages, it is the intangible that makes it useful.' After his death, his thoughts and ideas created one of the major branches in Chinese philosophy known to this day as Taoism.

The third book that is worth noting for its historical application of yin and yang, particularly in the realm of healing and early medicine, is the *Nei Ching*, otherwise known as the *Yellow Emperor's Classic of Internal Medicine*. This great treatise explains the intimate connection between a human being and his or her environment – the effect of cold, wind, heat on the well-being of the individual. The Yellow Emperor touches on the importance of living in harmony with nature, living with the seasons, eating what is growing at that time of year and what is local. He points out that good health and longevity is about adapting ourselves to the changes that occur in nature.

THE DYNAMICS OF YIN AND YANG

The original and traditional interpretation of yin and yang was that they represented the forces of earth and heaven (infinity). All life was seen to be influenced by these two opposite forces of energy generated by nature and the universe. Heaven's influence was yang, the earth's was yin – and the space between was inhabited by us. The concept implies that humanity and the natural world are charged by these two forces.

Using this fundamental model you can see that yang's basic energy descends. This downward force concentrates its power and speeds up towards the end of its cycle. You could therefore say that yang is a downward force that becomes more concentrated, harder, faster and generates more heat and activity as it pushes down. On the other hand, the expression of yin is an upward motion, emanating from the earth and returning to infinity. In this process yin will create a more expansive, diffuse quality, slowing down in the process, becoming cooler, softer and lighter.

The natural forces of yin and yang are therefore present in the constitutional structure of phenomena in the natural world. Both are likely to be present in differing amounts. Take for example a plant – its roots are a representation of yang's influence as they descend in search of water and nutrients, whereas the branches and the leaves are driven by yin's expansive, upward growing tendency. Later, when we look at our own constitutional make-up, we will be looking at how much of these yin/yang qualities were present at the time of our growth. For example, if you compare a spring onion with a carrot you will notice that the spring onion has far more upward growth than root. Conversely, the carrot is mainly root with a much lighter leaf structure above. In comparison you could say that the carrot has more yang in its structure than the spring onion, making it by comparison a more yang vegetable. The spring onion, driven by the upward rising force of yin with very little root structure, is undoubtedly more yin.

Structures that are harder and more concentrated have more yang than structures that are softer and lighter. For example, rocks and minerals that have taken time, pressure and fire to create are infinitely more yang than mushrooms that take a very little time to grow and are soft, expansive and here today gone tomorrow. It is interesting to note that aspects of these strong yang mineral qualities have formed the basis of our civilizations for the past 10,000 years – salt, coal, gold, diamonds and oil. It has been this yang foundation and not the commodities of water, fruit juice, vegetables and wood that have been the cornerstone of wealthy nations.

Later, in Chapter 3, we can begin to look at our condition in terms of yin and yang. Essentially, if we are hyperactive, self-motivated, fast or impatient, these are yang qualities. Conversely, if we are unenthusiastic, slow, tired, indifferent and need the support of others, these are fundamentally yang qualities. In nature an example of yin/yang qualities that you can observe on the plains lies in the lifestyle of the cheetah compared to its prey – a Thomson's gazelle. The yang qualities that the cheetah represents are its speed, intensity, that it generally hunts alone – whereas the Thomson's gazelle lives in a herd, is slower, needs to graze or feed more regularly. We all know 'yang' friends who can work hard and actively all day and just take one meal and be satisfied, while a more yin person may need to snack or eat or browse on a regular basis throughout the day.

It is important to remember that nothing is totally yang or totally yin. Both qualities need to be present within varying degrees. Nor is there any such thing as total balance where yin and yang are in complete equilibrium. If this occurred there would be no dynamism, therefore no action, no life. When we label something yin or yang what we are really saying is that there is a preponderance toward yin or yang within that structure or activity. The more extreme the presence of yin or yang within any structure, the greater the likelihood that its opposite is present in a smaller but equally dynamic proportion. For example, the harder and the more impregnable the shell of a nut may appear, the sweeter, softer or more delicious the kernel within. The ferocious highly active and protective and hard working bee can hide and produce the most delicious sweet (yin) honey.

Another quality of yin and yang that is worth understanding is that in their extreme forms both yin and yang become their opposite. If you take a glass of water and apply extreme amounts of yin to it – cold – it will eventually freeze and become harder (yang). That same water, when you apply large amount of yang (heat), will boil and eventually diffuse into steam and vapour. If you plunge into an icy cold bath in the morning, which is fundamentally yin, you are unlikely to leap out of the bath feeling yin for the manifestation of yin in this respect would be to feel relaxed, comfortable, sleepy. Far from this, the experience of strong yin will yangize you immediately. But if you were to take a hot (yang) bath it is unlikely that you would get out of it feeling invigorated, sharp, focused and hyperactive. Rocks and minerals under enormous pressure will eventually diffuse into either powder or liquid. The rising vapours from the earth eventually transform into rain, snow or hail and descend back to earth.

But apart from the obvious extremes, it is generally acknowledged that yin will create yin and yang will create yang. If you take the example of military life, which has a primarily yang function – discipline, defence, action and the use of fire and weapons – military commanders would need to bring a higher proportion of yang to the troops. They would be encouraged to get up early, take a run, take a cold shower, be precise in their timing and discipline, and eat simply at regular intervals. The Sergeant Major is highly unlikely to wake the soldiers at around 9 a.m. and ask whether they would like breakfast in bed, a long, hot bath and perhaps when they are ready could he see them on the parade ground! Although there is an obvious bias here towards yang there is one aspect that is yin – namely that soldiers of whatever rank obey orders and are fundamentally led. An example of a more potentially yin lifestyle could be that of a creative individual such as an artist, an author or a poet. Such a person needs space and time to be creative and the inspiration may occur at any time of day and night. Their friends and family may regard them as yin – they may work late into the night, they may prefer to get up later in the morning and their creativity may appear to come in bursts. All of this may appear essentially yin but there is one hidden yang essential factor: to be successful such people need to be self-motivated and their own leader.

EXAMPLES OF YIN AND YANG

Here are a few examples of yin and yang related to activity, work, the weather and foods. These are intended to give you some insight and 'muscle' as you begin to play with these concepts. Yin and yang thinking provides the backbone for assessing yourself, your current state of health and the game plan you will design in the following chapters. You can apply these observations and principles to every aspect to your life and these few examples serve as a taster.

Examples of yinizing activities can include dancing, yoga, swimming, receiving a massage, socializing, talking, passively observing sport, ballet or theatre. A good observation to make is that when we are feeling more yin we are more likely to be attracted to yin forms of entertainment and activity. We like to eat out and are happy to share ideas, our emotions and our thoughts with others. We are comfortable with the slow pace of activity with no limitations or time constraints. However, if we are feeling yang we are likely to feel impatient and irritated by recreational activity that has no apparent structure and is flowing along spontaneously. An excellent contemporary description of yin activities is to 'chill out' (yinize).

A short, sharp game of squash can be very yangizing, particularly if it has a competitive edge. If you are determined to win and improve your position within the club, then these factors combine to make it even more yang. One-to-one competitive sports are more demanding and yangizing than team sports where the focus of attention is not on you for the whole game. Golf, a popular sport nowadays for relaxation, is regarded by many as a means of getting away from the office or home, being in the open air, wandering for a few hours around expansive open spaces. In fact, it is a game which demands great accuracy, focus and a competitive edge – as does serious darts playing – both examples of yangizing sports.

Yin activities:	Yang activities:
• relaxing	• generate heat
• calming	• make you sweat
• intellectual	• are physical
• passive	• aggressive
• social	• fast
• trivial	• competitive
• gentle	• involve accuracy
• self-indulgent	• focusing (intense)

Work

People engaged in more yin activities where sensitivity and creativity are their most powerful assets undoubtedly feel uncomfortable when demands are made on them by their bosses regarding deadlines and final details. At a meeting of designers and artists at a major advertising agency, ideas and creativity may flow freely in a 30-minute conversation. The brilliant minds throw ideas around with such speed and agility that it is hard to keep track of the drift. But towards the end of the meeting, a big yang may make its presence felt in the shape of the financial director who grounds the whole conversation in terms of demanding detail, deadlines – who would be responsible for each area and when will the package be ready for approval? The highly charged creative atmosphere turns to one of stilted conversation. The yin creative minds don't have this skill and in the end the yang director will have to map out the deadlines and give them guidance on the nuts and the bolts of the project. He is like a bottle and they its contents which, like champagne, had exploded forth and now face the impossibly tricky task of trying to contain it back into the bottle.

If, on the other hand, your work is generally yangizing due to responsibility, attention to detail and having to meet deadlines, or if the work involves heavy physical labour, then you will need to balance this with some form of powerful yin. Generally, the harder people work and the more pressure they take the greater their desire to let off steam or to take on board yin to balance the situation. Early Friday evening, close to the major financial institutions in the big cities you will find masses of people pouring into clubs and bars to unwind over a drink. On my travels, whenever I worked as a labourer and was paid cash on a Friday afternoon, it was inevitable that we would all let our hair down on our way home. This could involve far too many drinks, a late night spicy meal in a Chinese or Indian restaurant or losing some of your hard-earned cash through betting. I always noticed that the hardest working, most yang individuals were inevitably broke again by Monday morning, and had usually spent their money on drinking, eating or gambling.

Yin:	Yang:
• creativity	• responsibility
• concepts	• leadership
• ideas	• attention to detail
• being supervized	• meeting deadlines
• little or no responsibility	• demanding of the nervous system
• sedentary	• physically demanding

Weather

Bear in mind the dynamics of yin and yang – that essentially yin creates yin and yang creates yang; but that in their extremes they create the opposite. It follows that moderately 'yang' climatic and weather conditions are going to make us feel more active, warm and outgoing. However, in their extreme they are likely to make us lazy and completely relaxed. Hence the tendency for inhabitants of colder, damper climates to enjoy holidays in the tropics. While 'yin' climatic conditions can make us more passive, less eager to dash about and more introverted, it is the extremes of these conditions that can bring about great burst of activity. The extremes of cold can produce some of the most demanding and physically active of sports. These can include skiing, ski jumping, ice hockey and rally driving – which demands great focus and co-ordination from our nervous system.

Yin weather:	Yang weather:
• humid/damp	• dry
• cold	• hot
• still	• stormy

Foods

I will go into this area in far more detail later but here are a few guidelines to determine some of the fundamental qualities. In looking at food you have to assess many factors, including the climate in which it grew, its nutritional make-up, whether it is animal or vegetable in origin and, most importantly, how it was cooked.

Yin foods include:	Yang foods include:
• cold foods	• hot or warm foods (soups and stews)
• sweet or spicy taste	• salty/savoury foods
• soft creamy texture	• dry texture
• very short cooking time	• foods that take time to cook
• vegetable quality food	• animal foods

Yin cooking styles:	Yang cooking styles:
• raw food	• roasting
• steaming	• baking
• blanching	• deep frying
• lightly fermented foods (yoghurt and beer)	• pressure cooking

You will notice that the inhabitants of the colder yin environments of the world have traditionally balanced this by eating predominantly from the yang examples that I have listed above. They are far more likely to enjoy a hot breakfast, plenty of soups and stews, well cooked foods such as breads and cakes, smoked foods, salted foods and especially roasted animal products. Whereas in the warmer, more yang tropical regions of the world the inhabitants are far more likely to enjoy spicy foods, softer foods, cooler foods such as fruits and salads and have a higher intake of vegetable foods in the shape of grain and bean rather than meat and baked flour products.

3

Understanding Ourselves

We have seen how before undertaking any voyage, you would need to establish the kind of vessel you would be using. For example, a sailing boat or a motor cruiser. You would also need to investigate the current condition of the craft: the state of the engine, how much fuel, water and food on board?

In understanding ourselves relative to any change we wish to undertake, our constitution relates to the capacity and potential that we are born into. This is given us by our parents and manifests in our structure, which is unlikely to change during the course of our lives. Our condition is a different matter altogether. This is in a constant mode of change from active to passive, tired or energetic, overweight or underweight, happy or sad.

Another way of helping to distinguish the difference between constitution and condition would be to look at a piece of wooden furniture. Its basic structure, the materials that it was made of, essentially define its constitution. The qualities that are present within its construction and design are unlikely to be capable of change, for example, your dining-room table may be made of oak, maybe two metres by one. It cannot change overnight into beech or pine wood nor is it likely to expand or shrink in any dramatic way. However, its condition can change. It could become scratched, dirty, polished, mouldy or cracked and dry. The constitution of a table made of hardwood (yang) – oak or beech – is more robust, more contracted and can withstand more use and pressure. A table built of softer (yin) material such as pine is far more likely to scratch or dent, and less likely to withstand the ravages of frequent heavy use.

UNDERSTANDING OUR CONSTITUTION

By being able to define our unique constitution we are better able to understand where our potential strengths and weaknesses lie. It is then a lot easier to decide what kind of route to take in life in order to take advantage of inherent strengths. If you choose the opposite approach, the added challenge can undoubtedly, in the long term, be potentially a rewarding and enlightening experience. However, the path of least resistance is ultimately the easiest route to take.

Our constitution is revealed to us by the aspects of our physical make-up that are inherently unchanging. Essentially these are our bone structure and our size. In this chapter we consider the shape and size of our head, our hands or feet, the shape and size of our ears and our teeth. In constitution yang can be defined as robust, practical and steady. Yin constitutional qualities would be revealed in taller or thinner bone structures demonstrating a more delicate, intellectual and changeable nature. Neither should be regarded as good or bad, but understanding who we are constitutionally can help us to take advantage of this potential and use it creatively in our lives.

Yin/yang structure

Look at your own constitutional structure, observing your body shape, face shape, the shape of your hands and fingers, your teeth, ears and eyebrows. Yin and yang provide us with the underlying models for this observation and as a reminder here are some of the qualities of yin and yang in the table below:

Yin	Yang
• expansion	• contraction
• dispersing	• gathering
• vertical	• horizontal
• thinner	• thicker
• bigger	• smaller
• delicate	• durable

Body shape

Look at your basic physical structure in comparison with other people of your generation and race. Generally, the taller and thinner and more fine your bone structure the more yin your constitution. However, if you are shorter, stockier and have big bones you are fundamentally yang in constitution. Western people have become taller in the past two generations and undoubtedly this is due to the increased intake of yin quality foods such as milk and sugar-based products. In Japan, after World War II, dairy products, sugar and confectionery became a part of the Japanese diet. Children born after 1955 are on average 12 cm (5 inches) taller than their parents or grandparents. In Central Africa, the Tutsi and Hutu people are amongst the tallest in the world. Their main source of sustenance is derived from the rearing of cattle and the use of their by-products – especially milk products. It is curious to note that in Central Africa, near neighbours of the Tutsi and Hutu people were the pygmies – the smallest and most yang constitutionally structured people in the world. Unlike their neighbours who inhabit a more open environment, the pygmy people were forest dwellers. Wild meat, wild berries, wild vegetables and tubers – all essentially yang products – form the basis of their traditional diet.

One of the main sources of good quality yang in the diet of our ancestors was minerals. There are two ways of ensuring a good intake and absorption of the minerals found in food. Firstly, it is important to eat foods that are rich in minerals and secondly it is wise to reduce or avoid foods that have a tendency to de-mineralize the body. A good source of minerals in a traditional diet would have been in the skins and leaves of vegetables, the skin and the bone of fish, poultry or meat. During my travels around the world in my twenties, I shared endless meals in Third World countries with a whole family seated together. If grandma or grandad were at the table you would notice them eat every scrap on the plate and chew their food really well. In Malaysia or in Indonesia when you ate small sea or lake fish you would eat the whole fish including the bones and skin. I have eaten chicken in Laos where we ate every part of the bird including the head, the beak and the feet. I remembered being offered the well-boiled beak in my portion of the meal as it represented to my hosts a delicacy. In reality it was providing me with the richest source of mineral. In the West two generations ago it was not uncommon for families to eat cooked meat offal, and stews and soups that had a basis of animal bone. Nowadays the preference is for filleted meat and softer white meat flesh such as chicken breast. Where, traditionally, root vegetables such as carrots, would only be scrubbed, we now peel them, remove the tap root, remove the green tops and eat the softer part from within. Although these are only general examples, it is important to remember that our general development in terms of constitution is undoubtedly heading towards a yin phase.

Another feature of our body structure to observe is the size of the head in relation to the body. It is not only relevant to note whether you are tall or short but also whether your head is relatively big or small in proportion to your body. A large head is a more yang constitutional trait. A smaller head in relation to a larger body is more yin.

Face shape

A further piece in the puzzle of your constitutional nature is the shape of your face. If your head is more thin, narrow, oval or triangular, with the point of the triangle towards your chin and the broader aspect at the forehead, this is a yin face shape. A square or round head or a triangular shaped head with the base at jaw level are all signs of a yang constitution. Where the features appear more delicate – this is yin – or where the features of your face appear robust – this is more yang. Using the yin/yang model of expansion and contraction, you can then look more closely at the features of the face. A general contraction of these features such as a smaller mouth, a narrower nose and eyes set closer together are an indication of yang whereas the dispersing quality of yin could manifest as bigger eyes, further apart, broader nose and a wider mouth.

Hands

Our hands can reveal a lot of information about our constitutional potential. Remember that the definition of yang in this context is in connection with our practical, pragmatic nature; the yin is associated with our artistic, intuitive nature. Thick fleshy hands (yang) manifest in a powerful, practical nature as well as the potential for this individual to have vitality and stamina. Thin, delicate hands would represent an artistic nature, a more intellectual approach to life and more of a tendency to depend on intuition. Square palms (yang) indicate a grounded nature whereas yin qualities such as adaptability and a sense of vision are more likely to be represented in longer shaped palms. The best way to judge whether your palms are square or more elongated is to measure the distance between the base of the fingers and the base of the wrist and compare it with the overall width of the palm. If both measurements are closely matched this is a square palm. There are many studies related to the lines of the palm with which we are born, and traditional cultures associate them with not only our constitution but our destiny. In practical terms, lines on the hand that appear deep, clear and without any diversions would constitute a yang palm indicating a straightforward life. However, lines that are more superficial, that are not clearly defined but that tend to diverge or 'fray' indicate a lack of stability and many changes in life.

The palm of our hand can represent our physical nature – our practical capacity, our physical strength and stamina, whereas our fingers can represent our mind, our spirituality and our thinking. Long, delicate fingers (yin) represent a mind full of ideas, vision and intuition. Short, thick and stubby fingers are much more likely to show a tendency toward careful measure thinking and practical down-to-earth thinking. Straight fingers, whether they are long or short, would represent a more straightforward mind – capable of staying with the subject or staying focused in one domain. Fingers that bend towards the side represent a tendency for the person to think or approach the problem in many different ways. This can be a useful attribute in certain situations, but it can lead to a more scattered way of thinking as well. Whether your fingers are long or short, check whether they are well padded with flesh. If you hold your fingers closely together and raise them towards a light, see if any gaps appear. If your fingers are well-clad with flesh you are unlikely to see any gaps and this is an indication that you received good nourishment in embryo which essentially leaves you with a stronger constitution. 'Thinner' fingers are an indication of a lack of some nutrients while in embryo – particularly minerals – which in turn can lead to a more delicate constitution.

Always remember that at this stage of your observations you are looking at the constitutional features – those qualities that you are born with and that are unlikely to change – rather than conditional qualities – whether your hands are damp or dry – which are connected with your current condition and as a result is in a continual state of change.

Teeth

Our teeth, like our bones, provide a very good gauge to the strength of our constitution. Both are the product of our family's nutrition, especially the quantity and diversity of minerals. It always amazed me when I travelled in Third World countries how strong and healthy people's teeth were in comparison with the West. Teeth would be used for a variety of tasks that would make most Westerners shudder. Even elderly folk would have no difficulty cracking the bones of a chicken; others would crack open the toughest nutshells with their teeth, and most awesome use of the teeth that I observed was opening a bottle of beer or Coca Cola. Smaller teeth are yang whereas larger teeth are yin; teeth that grow closely together are more yang whereas those that have a tendency to gaps between them are more yin. Teeth that grow inwards have a yang attribute whereas teeth that point slightly outwards or towards the front have a yin tendency. These three yin/yang categories are essentially associated with our parents – particularly our mother's – diet. The yang factors in their development include plenty of minerals, salt, animal food and the yin factors include higher intakes of carbohydrates, fats or sugars.

Ears

Like our fingerprints our ears are quite unique and represent much about our constitutional make-up. In oriental medicine they are seen as a microcosm of the body and there is a system of acupuncture that treats only points found on the ear. The ear is seen as a miniature version of the embryo, the head represented in the lobe, the spine on the outside ridge of the ear and the internal organs positioned around the entrance to the ear itself. Overall, the bigger your ears and the fleshier they appear the more robust your physical constitution. Smaller ears that lack a lobe indicate a more delicate physical constitution. It has been my observation that ears appear to be getting smaller by the generation. You only have to sit in a market square or bar in any part of Europe to see fairly small elderly people with large fleshy ears and well-formed ear lobes. Large ears are also a sign of slower and steadier metabolism, whereas the small ear can represent someone who is faster, quicker and has a tendency to burn out quickly.

Ears, naturally, can tell us a lot about a person's capacity to 'listen'. The bigger your ears, the more you are going to hear. Ears that are flat against the head will hear sounds from all directions, whereas ears that protrude away from the head are likely to hear from a limited direction. The best listeners therefore are people with large ears that lie close to their head. One of my favourite studies of this area is looking at photographs of traditional North American Indian chiefs. They all had very large ears sitting close to the head. Many judges, rulers and military leaders also have large, fleshy ears. A good example of ears can be found in that very British institution – the House of Lords. Many are the descendants of former politicians, governors or military leaders and their function is to listen and to give their judgement on the House of Commons.

Conclusion

Any aspect of our physical make-up with which we were born and that is essentially unchanging can be used to assess our potential and capacity. I have given just a few examples of this exciting insight and if you wish to develop your skills further then I encourage you to watch and watch and watch! There are people all around you; television provides many examples and newspapers and magazines are another great source of study. The purpose of bringing this material into the programme is to give you a sense of your own nature and that in turn helps you to reflect on whether you are either challenging your potential or matching it. For example, if your constitution reveals that you are an ideas person or an innovator then you will undoubtedly feel stuck and uncomfortable in a job where you are completing tasks for someone else. Ideally you are best matched in a position where your creativity is utilized. However, on a more philosophical note, you might decide to try and develop patience or understanding by forcing yourself to listen to and complete the works of others. It is up to you to decide!

UNDERSTANDING OUR CONDITION

Whereas constitution is impossible to alter since it is derived form the structure that we are born with, giving us our essential potential and capacity in life, our condition is well within our scope for change. Condition can be defined as how we feel on a day-to-day, hour-to-hour level and it is in a constant state of flux. Given that it has this potential, we have a lot of say in how we feel as we can control the various factors that affect our health. By understanding these factors that fuel our condition we can begin to remove some extremes that may be upsetting our equilibrium.

In the Orient, they consider that the absorption of food, liquid, air and Chi make up our current condition. Food is about our daily diet, finding a balance that is suitable for our condition and our activity. It is important here that the 'fuel' suits both our nature and our lifestyle. Excess is the cause of many health imbalances. Liquid can be defined as our daily fluid, the quality of water that we drink, whether our drinks are hot or cold, and that the volume of fluid that we take in is appropriate to our metabolism. Air is about our capacity to exercise and oxygenate well. It is also reflected in the quality of air we breathe as this has a major impact on our health. Although the word Chi can be translated from the Chinese to mean literally spirit, the same word is used in Japan but called Ki, in India this energy is Prana and in ancient Egypt Kaa. In English, we could describe this Chi as life force or spirit. It is an intangible force that provides the dynamic in the natural world and is responsible for our vitality.

A simple way to determine how important these factors are is to ask the question – how long can you survive without any of them? A healthy individual could probably survive without food thirty to forty days; but we would suffer severe dehydration and potential kidney failure if we did not take in any fluid for six or seven days. Without air, we can come unstuck in two to three minutes and are usually brain-dead after six to seven minutes. But how long without Chi? Given that this is our basic life force, our spirit, we need this factor more than the previous three. Without Chi we have no life. Rather than surviving for weeks or days or minutes, we can probably survive only seconds or milliseconds without Chi!

A large proportion of the body is made up of fluid, so much so that just over half of our body mass is essentially liquid based. When the body is cremated, the residual ashes and bone can easily fit inside a shoebox. Already you can see that the essential 'mass' of a human being is relatively small in comparison to our living and dynamic structure. However, you could take this process one step further. Our inner core, our bone structure, is made up of billions of atoms and molecules. These in turn are made up of protons, neutrons and electrons which are moving within space within these so-called molecules. Although impossible to do at this stage, imagine that you were able to remove the 'space' within each molecule and compress the residual mass of protons, neutrons and electrons. Compress this total mass and the question now is – how big is a human being? The answer is about the size of a match head! This begs the question what is a human being? A simple answer would be that we are little more than physicalized Chi or spirit. In other words, what keeps us alive and physical is determined by our absorption of food, liquid, air and Chi. When we cease to absorb these factors, we die and return to Chi – or spirit. Assessing and understanding the levels and quality of our input of these four vital factors plays the single most important role in determining our health and current condition.

The effect of Chi

Although Chi is invisible and intangible, it has very similar qualities to water. The quality and freshness of water is largely dependent on how much oxygen is present. When Chi is not vibrant, it brings with it a feeling of heaviness, darkness and dampness. Chi that is bright appears warm, refreshing and light. All of us have the capacity to intuitively sense Chi. For example, if we greet an old friend that we haven't seen for several months it is very easy in the initial few minutes to perceive their Chi. Do they seem happy or sad? Are they burdened or full of the joys of spring? All of us have walked into a room where two people have been engaged in a disagreement or argument and, although they stopped the discussion on our entry, we could feel or sense the Chi in the atmosphere. When we go house or flat-hunting we are inevitably aware of the home's Chi. Initially, we may have been attracted to it for economic or location reasons. However, these more rational thoughts are put on hold as we switch to a more intuitive mode. It is often hard to qualify what we feel or perceive. We say: 'I like the feel of this place,' or 'it feels spooky,' or 'I like the energy here.' When our own Chi is blocked we see little to be optimistic about; we also feel that everything that we are undertaking is an effort. If, on the other hand, our Chi is highly-charged our enthusiasm and exuberance can be likened to a young puppy on a leash – straining to get away to explore new horizons.

Two kinds of Chi effect us. The first I call universal Chi which essentially is raining down on all of us but will influence us in different ways. We have little or no control over this kind of Chi. It manifests itself through the seasons, the weather, the time of day or major international events. The second kind of Chi I call individual Chi. It is through this that we are directly influenced, by Chi from our environment, our work or relationships, and essentially we are partly responsible for it and could, if we wished, begin to deflect this Chi or change the manner in which we cope with it.

A good example of universal Chi is the season of the year. If you live in a temperate climate that enjoys four seasons, you are likely to be affected by the change of energy that is present as you move from season to season. It is quite natural in the depths of winter to feel lower in Chi than at other times, and this is quite noticeable in the surrounding natural environment. You don't see the grass grow; the leaves have disappeared from the trees; most of the bird life has migrated and many wild mammals are quietly hibernating. It is our natural tendency during the winter months to hibernate our Chi and feel less enthusiastic about initiating new ideas, staying out late or driving overnight for a weekend away. The Chi of spring naturally brings with it a feeling of freshness, aliveness and frequently a desire to shake off the cobwebs of winter. Traditional, we would use this time to spring clean. The Chi of summer brings with its warmth the desire to socialize more, to relax, to travel and perhaps to put in longer hours on work or projects. The natural environment is in full bloom and in reflecting this we can also be more animated and sociable. The autumn brings with it the opportunity to gather our Chi, to become a little more introspective, perhaps begin to study on an evening course or to take stock of our financial situation. Nature is also consolidating and yangizing at this time of year and this process is important to all of us as we prepare for the lower levels of Chi that will be available to us universally during the winter months ahead. A healthy, flexible condition allows us to adapt to these seasons, whereas if our condition is stuck we inevitably feel overburdened by the current season. Either it is too hot or the nights are too long or we do not have the energy to adapt to change and new projects.

Another form of universal Chi that inevitably plays a part in how we feel and our condition is the weather. We have no control over this Chi but how we adapt or react to it is very much related to our condition. Even the sunniest, brightest day of the summer can seemingly have little or no uplifting effect on someone whose condition is profoundly stuck. On the other hand, a damp, windy, drizzly day seems to have little or no effect on the bright Chi of young children as they play outside oblivious to the elements. We can all relate to how we feel on a Monday morning, when the heavens open and the effect of this Chi on us just adds to the pressure or despondency of having to go to work. You only have to experience flying from a damp, four seasons climate in mid-winter to a warm holiday in the sunshine to notice the effect of this kind of Chi on you. It is equally obvious when you return to the damp and the cold how the weather manifests in the Chi of people's body language and expression. We often don't notice the effect of this universal Chi as we live with it all the time; it is only when we are objective about it that it becomes more obvious.

The time of day also affects our Chi. The energy of dawn brings with it the feeling of newness and growth which, if we are up early enough, we can experience. By getting up later we miss out on this natural change and it can lead to an inevitable feeling of despondency and gloom. The Chi is at its most fiery at midday. Here we have the potential to harness the qualities of clear communication and activity. Everybody's Chi naturally starts to sink and settle in the afternoon, and it is not uncommon that offices and factories take a break around 3 p.m. and attempt to restore their employees' Chi with a hot drink and a sweet snack. In many parts of the world, this sinking form of Chi is reflected in people's desire to take a siesta. A short rest like this, in tune with the day's Chi, can be very refreshing and fits neatly with the cycle of Chi through a 24-hour period. Around sunset and into the early evening our Chi can begin to gather and we draw in energy by returning home or attending an evening class. If you combine the Chi of both winter and the evening you are far more likely to feel like going home rather than socialize or go to a party. However, an evening in the summer may well find you away from home. The Chi of the night is quiet and still and has the effect of recharging and stabilizing our condition. Working through the night can disrupt this pattern as can eating late in the evening or retiring well after midnight. The Yellow Emperor, in the *Nei Ching*, points out that the secret to good health and longevity is to live in harmony with the seasons and the cycles of the day.

International events can also affect our universal Chi. In times of war or economic pressure everyone feels the effect. Even small children who are unaware of the details of what is occurring, inevitably pick up from adults a sense of unease or worry. Famine and drought equally affect everybody's Chi, another example of a quality of Chi over which we have no control. An international event, such as a major football match between two countries, can influence the Chi of the nation for a few hours.

We are all consciously or unconsciously aware of the Chi that we pick up from our work, our work environment, our colleagues, our home, our relationships, our neighbours and relatives. When our own Chi is low or vulnerable we are far more likely to be affected by these external factors, far more than when our Chi is bright and direct. Have you ever noticed that when you are tired or despondent you seem to attract what I call a 'Chi vampire'? These are seemingly friendly people who have the habit of telephoning or calling in at a time when your Chi is vulnerable, and they seem to have the effect of draining your last few remaining grams of Chi! Is it not curious to note that they don't telephone or show up when your Chi is bright? On the other hand, some people have remarkably strong Chi that can invigorate and inspire you when you feel at a low ebb. Provided they are in good health, you are not draining them by being inspired by them – they simply provide a great tonic for you at that time. Being around individuals who constantly complain, are frequently irritable or have an air of hopelessness about their lives, inevitably rubs off on you to a greater or lesser extent. Have you ever noticed the effect when you do not feel particularly well but someone says, 'You look well today!' It seems to lift your spirits, gives you a boost and inevitably you can begin to live into that new feeling of improvement. If, however, when you feel low in energy and someone says, 'You look tired today,' the effect can be equally profound but in the opposite direction. It emphasizes, and in many ways, exaggerates your feelings of lethargy and tiredness. Being criticized or encouraged both affect our Chi. Finding a rewarding new job or losing one, debts, winning a lottery, celebrating a birthday or attending a funeral all affect our Chi.

A major factor in our current lifestyle is the effect of so-called 'stress'. When you examine stress it is obvious that it has no physicality, it is more a state of being. Why is it then that some situations that are stressful to some seem an inspiration to someone else? It is our capacity and flexibility to deal with change and pressure that leads to the symptoms of stress. If our Chi is clear and bright we attract a lot of activity and do not feel any pressure from the additional work. However, when our Chi is low any kind of pressure can seem daunting and can lead us into feelings of despondency and despair. Since life itself is a dynamic between action and rest, we need to apply the same principle regarding work. To balance all our manual work we need recreational activities that are physically relaxing but stimulate our mind. If we are under enormous cerebral pressure at work our recreational activity needs to be physical and less demanding on our nervous system. By beginning to understand our condition we can be better prepared to balance this with activities and work that both stimulate and relax our condition. Too much of the same – all work and no play – will inevitably lead to physical and emotional stress as well as create unnecessary pressure in our home lives. Ultimately, it is our choice how we choose to work and how we choose to live.

One area where Chi can effect us profoundly is in our relationships with other people. Whether it is because our partner is unhappy, our colleague at work is irritable, we are currently in dispute with our neighbour or we have lost touch with a close relative, it all effects our Chi. Although we may perceive the other person as the problem, that their attitude needs to change, we can begin to manifest change in ourselves by looking at how we are relating to them. Much of the negativity directed at us can be resolved through open communication. Even if this route seems impossible, it is possible to change your attitude or your

Chi towards the other person. A simple act of generating warm thoughts towards them, forgiveness and a willingness to accept them for who they are can begin to change the effect of Chi on you. But undoubtedly, face-to-face communication to help clarify any misunderstandings or negativity is the answer. In Chapter 8, you will find examples designed to redress this imbalance of Chi through forgiveness, letting go of resentment and dissolving old patterns of thinking and being.

The Chi that we receive from our home also plays a vital role in our health and in our condition. As the space that we use to regroup our energy and nourish ourselves our home is essentially our springboard into the world. The Chinese have a fascinating system known as Feng Shui which is considered to be both an art and a science that can benefit the occupants of homes and other buildings. Much of what is practised in Feng Shui is pure common-sense. It is also fundamentally based on an understanding of Chi and how it affects and pervades the space in which you live. Chi, which moves in both the landscape and the home environment in a way similar to water, needs to flow freely in order to be vital. When Chi is blocked it can bring about stagnation; when Chi is uncontrolled it can bring confusion and disorder. Feng Shui and oriental healing systems have one major objective in common – they are essentially to do with prevention. In traditional times people would give considerable thought and planning to where they placed their homes so that they could benefit best from the landscape's Chi. Planning the location, position and design of your home to allow a beneficial circulation of Chi will undoubtedly enhance the well-being of the occupants. However, in the West we tend to plan and build our homes and offices along economic lines rather than considering the effect of Chi within the building. In much the same way Western medicine spends a very small proportion of the funds available on prevention. Most resources are used in the acute stage. In some traditions of Chinese medicine it remains common to pay your doctor to keep you well and withhold payment when you become ill!

Without turning this book into a Feng Shui manual, here are a few common-sense points that we can benefit from understanding. Rather than see these as conclusions or simple 'fix-its', try to understand the system from a Chi point of view. The neighbourhood that you live in plays a big part in the Chi that you receive from your environment. Does the area have a high crime rate or a relatively low one? Is your locality favoured by retired people or by families with young children? The Chi of your neighbours undoubtedly rubs off on how you feel and the potential that you derive from your locality. Roads can be symbolic of rivers which in turn reflect how Chi moves. If you live very close to a main, busy road then you are likely to feel influenced by the constant movement, the busy-ness of the location, and undoubtedly feel distracted as a result. On the other hand, you may live in a quiet cul-de-sac where Chi enters from a main road but has no way of finding a natural exit. The Chi will naturally dam up in the cul-de-sac and pace of life, as a result, will be slow, bordering on stagnant. Natural and man-made objects that stand within 300 metres (100 ft) of your property can have the effect of what the Chinese call 'cutting Chi'. This means that lamp posts, telegraph poles, electricity pylons, large trees can direct their energy like a knife-edge towards your property and the effect is like that of being attacked. Tall buildings close by can act as a safe protection but they can also overshadow you and result in a feeling of being threatened. Cutting Chi can be deflected by using shutters on your windows or by other methods that I describe further in Chapter 8.

The entrance to your home is very important. This is the mouth into which Chi enters the body of the house. Notice whether your hallway is cluttered with shoes, walking sticks, umbrellas, coats or a telephone table piled up with magazines and mail. Is your entrance way narrow, dark and unwelcoming? Is your hallway clean, bright and welcoming? All of these factors affect how Chi enters the house and on a more subtle level begin to benefit the health and welfare of the occupants. Chi, like air, needs to circulate well in a healthy environment. Rooms that are dark or that lack proper ventilation or bright light from outside will naturally feel stagnant and you will find difficulty feeling inspired. You can use mirrors and lighting, plants and flowers to open up space that feels like this. In some household designs there is a through draught of Chi – this is where the front door opens into a hallway that leads to a room at the back of the house where there is a door or conservatory into the garden. On a windy day, with the back door open you know the effect of this syndrome. There is a gale of air rushing through the house – perhaps one of the doors slam. The effect of this 'rushing' Chi is that it can cause distraction and confusion and a lack of being able to see a project through to its completion. Somehow you need to dampen down and soften this rush of Chi so that opportunities do not come in one door and leave through the one opposite. Wind chimes were traditionally used for this role, carefully placed to break up and soften the violent flow of Chi through the house.

Old, negative or stagnant Chi has a habit of impregnating our environment at home. Soft furnishings such as bedding, curtains, carpets and drapes all have the capacity to absorb Chi from the atmosphere. Having these items replaced or cleaned frequently brings a sense of lightness and freshness into your environment. For this reason I would never consider buying a second-hand mattress as the previous owner's Chi will undoubtedly be absorbed. A few antiques in your home, passed down from relatives, can bring a certain sense of stability to the Chi of your home, but conversely filling your home with antiques or second-hand soft furnishing brings with it an air of stagnation. If you are always rushing around and have little stability in your life then perhaps a few well-placed objects that represent stability can help.

The Chi of the previous occupant of your home can also play a part on your health, wealth and well-being. Did their business go bankrupt? Was your flat occupied by a young woman who recently left to become married? Was your home previously occupied by a healthy family whose breadwinner moved on because of promotion? Did the previous occupant have failing health? What was the building that you occupy used for in the past – are you living in an apartment that used to be a church or a hospital or a slaughter house or stables for horses? All these factors can influence the Chi you feel in any building for either bad or good. Spring cleaning or holding a lively house-warming party are practical ways to break up some of this inherited stagnant Chi in your new home. The perception of Chi is not unique to oriental people. We all have the capacity to sense and feel space and I invite you to look at how you can balance and enhance the Chi within your own home and office.

The effect of oxygen

As with Chi, there are two considerations regarding the air that we breathe. You and I have little or no direct control over the quality of air that we receive from the environment. We are all dependent on the healthy process of photosynthesis from plants and trees to give us an abundant supply of oxygen. Environmental scientists are warning us that this quality is fast being eroded and that even if we were to begin to reverse the damage today, it would take some fifty years before the quality of air returned to where it was only ten years ago. Where we do have a choice, however, are in the areas of exercise, breathing techniques, fresh air, smoking and surrounding ourselves with good sources of oxygen such as plants.

Oxygen is a primary life force for all of us. When we have access to plenty through vigorous oxygenation by means of exercise or dancing, we feel light, charged and enthusiastic. If you were to take a break from sedentary work and take a quick, fast jog around the block you would inevitably return feeling breathless and perhaps slightly giggly as well. Higher levels of oxygen in the blood stream are well known to cause euphoria and laughter. On the other hand, when we do not receive enough oxygen we can feel heavy, tired and despondent. This heaviness of Chi can correspond to the emotion of depression. Literally, to feel depressed in this sense means a lack of oxygen. Seeing the world through a condition that is poorly oxygenated gives us a darker and bleaker outlook. A long walk in the fresh air can help sweep away these cobwebs and give us new clarity and new 'inspiration'.

Here are some areas that have a direct effect on our input of oxygen and I invite you to look at those where you could bring about a change. They are all practical, common-sense and easy to follow:

Physical exercise

Given that we all have unique constitutions and conditions there is no fixed formula. However, three vital areas of exercise need to be included in any programme for it to allow us to receive oxygen and good stimulation at the same time. Provided you are reasonably healthy and flexible, you need to design an exercise programme that you enjoy and perform it at least three times a week for approximately twenty minutes. The first component that you need to build into this programme is the capacity to generate sweat during oxygenation. Sweating is one of the body's methods of eliminating excess fluids and toxins from the system. On a daily basis we all loose half a litre (nearly a pint) of fluid through our breath and sweat. This volume of liquid naturally rises the harder we exercise and the more we sweat.

Secondly, we need to become breathless during our exercise programme. This not only strengthens the muscles in our chest but also expands the lungs to their full capacity and helps us to use a bigger area of our lungs even when we are sedentary. Our lung capacity is about 7.7 litres (1.7 gallons), and the interior surface area of our lungs is twenty-five times the surface area of our entire skin. By exercising and getting breathless we can open up this potential and release any stagnation (through coughing) that may have built up. The third component that is essential in any exercise programme is excitement. By stimulating the adrenal glands through danger or pressure, we begin to unwind tension that may be building up within our nervous system, our lungs and other vital organs. The best way to design this component is to find some form of exercise that becomes a challenge. I used to go to a gym three times a week and found that I could sweat and become breathless very easily but the experience was not challenging or exciting. Exercise such as horseback riding, mountain biking, team and competitive sports can provide all three important components.

Breathing techniques

Meditation, martial arts, yoga, Chi Kung, Shiatsu and Tai Chi all have one common denominator in terms of their fundamental discipline – breathing. Chi and air are closely linked and it is by harnessing these two factors that the true power of any of these systems is obtained.

Where fresh air and exercise essentially improve our breathing capacity, focused breathing techniques add depth and power to our utilization of air. Next time you are in a hurry when walking, try this technique to improve your speed and stamina. While walking, draw a deep breath through your nose fairly quickly (2-3 seconds). Next, hold your breath for at least 4-5 seconds to allow this breath to be charged by Chi. Finally, breathe out through pursed lips for up to 8 seconds, pumping your breath out as if your lungs were a pair of powerful pistons. Also, while you breathe out, keep your focus and intention sharp on the purpose of your walk or destination. You will notice a surge in speed and strength as you breathe out.

Fresh air

Having a good supply of fresh air where we live, sleep and work is vital to our well-being. This is an area where you have a direct say in the matter. Since you spend some 6-9 hours a night sleeping, make sure that your room has a good circulation of fresh air. Provided security is not an issue it is good advice to sleep with your window slightly open. Traditional people, in whatever climate, would always fling open the windows daily to allow air to circulate and break up any stagnation that existed. Office environments are far more challenging as there are so many more people to consider. However, it is possible to request that people do not smoke or to share space with someone who also appreciates the quality of fresh air. If neither can be achieved, make sure that every ninety minutes you can go out on to a balcony or stroll outside, even if it is just for a few minutes. Many of us spend considerable time commuting to and from work every day. Try to find a method of transportation that gives you the best source of fresh air. This will find you reasonably refreshed when you arrive at work and equally can leave you with a greater sense of enthusiasm and energy when you return home.

Central heating and air-conditioning

These two marvellous luxuries of our modern lifestyle can also begin to weaken our condition and affect how we feel through the air that they provide for us. Make sure that in your home the central heating does not come on until you are awake in the morning, otherwise the hot and stuffy air inevitably leaves you feeling tired (yin) when you wake up. Excessive central heating undoubtedly has a yinizing effect on us all and the symptoms of this are tiredness, lethargy and a lack of drive. While the excessive heat in many countries leaves us feeling lethargic and yin, coolness helps to keep us fresh and alert and vital. During the British colonial era in India, this concept was well understood years before the development of air-conditioning. For the British to remain in control they needed to be essentially yang: focused, controlling, dominant, active and alert. During the hot season it was inevitable that everybody drooped and was lethargic. However, the British moved their regional seats of government during that season to six or seven locations in the mountains known as 'hill stations'. The higher altitude and the cooler temperature allowed them to continue the machinations of government unhindered by the hot weather.

One of the drawbacks of air-conditioning is the way in which many systems recycle air. This can lead to the transmission of viruses and has a general drying (yangizing) effect on the atmosphere. The second disadvantage to the perpetual use of air-conditioning in very hot parts of the world – in the home, the car and the office – is that it alienates the inhabitants from their local environment. This manifests as a lack of adaptability and a general weakening of the immune system. In the long run, it is far healthier to adapt to the climate and the seasons and, ideally, to design your home or office in ways that traditional people would have employed to cope with the oppressive heat.

Smoking

This is an area where undoubtedly you have a choice. You also have some choice in whether you wish to be around people who smoke at home or in the office. Luckily we are living in a culture that now respects your right to request a smoke-free zone. If you are a smoker, and you are considering this ten-day programme, then you might wish to stop smoking for the ten-day period as well! An added challenge! Here are a few well-known factors that could help determine your decision:

- It is important to realize that nicotine is not only absorbed in the lungs but is also absorbed directly into the bloodstream through the lining of the mouth. If you have been living with an argument that cigar or pipe smoking is safer do remember this.
- Nicotine is a poison. If you were to take orally the concentrated dose of nicotine found in twenty cigarettes you would be killed by the paralysis that nicotine would cause to your lungs.
- Seventy per cent of tar from cigarettes and tobacco remains in the airways and this tar has been known to develop cancer on living tissue.

- The smoking of tobacco increases the amount of carbon monoxide in the blood. Carbon monoxide is widely understood to be a major contributor to heart disease.
- The adrenal glands are directly stimulated by nicotine. This rise in adrenal activity can raise the blood pressure which brings with it the added risk of a stroke or consequent brain damage. Nicotine also has the habit of keeping fat in the bloodstream which in turn can build up and lead to other forms of heart and circulatory disease.

If you are a committed smoker, and you feel confident that you are not addicted, then prove this to yourself three or four times a year by giving it a break. This is a great way to exercise real freedom. Being able to start and stop when you please, not feeling agitated because you have run out of tobacco, would help prove that you are not dependent. However, few can manage this – and their health risks are still high.

Plants

From what we understand of evolution there was originally little or no oxygen in the atmosphere. It was green plants that began the process of photosynthesis whereby the sun's energy helped to break up water into hydrogen and oxygen. In the last billion years oxygen levels have slowly increased so that current levels in the atmosphere are about 20 per cent. So green plants on the planet are vital to our survival. Their main function is to return oxygen to the air. In terms of evolution we as human beings are relatively new. Of the mass of living creatures on the planet only 15 per cent live on the land, while the remainder draw their oxygen from the sea. When we take a look at the whole spectrum of evolution we can see that not only are we relatively new but also fairly vulnerable.

Healthy plants in our home and office environments help to charge the atmosphere. Fresh cut flowers can also help but nothing beats a living plant. I recommend the kind of plant that requires attention and that is more delicate. Dry, yang plants such as cacti are not going to do the same job in your home as those with vulnerable, soft growth. Take care of your plants as they reflect your health – especially that of your lungs. Begin to notice where they thrive better, what they respond to in terms of water, air and sunlight. Perhaps you can begin to introduce them into your office space but remember to take care of them.

The effect of liquid

Since our body is made up of some 60 per cent fluid in terms of volume, it is important that we recharge and maintain the balance of this on a daily basis. We have seen that without any physical exertion in a temperate climate we lose half a litre (close to a pint) of fluid every day simply in the process of respiration and mild sweating. Beyond this half litre, all of us need approximately 1½ to 2½ litres (2½ to 4½ pints) per day to recharge our fluid intake, to balance the electrolyte system and to replenish fluid in our blood and vital organs. If we take on a very small amount of liquid we soon become dehydrated, dry, withered and yang. Too much liquid and we are bloated, heavy, tired, lethargic and yin. A lot of people consider that they are overweight but a closer examination from an oriental perspective often reveals that they are simply overloaded with fluid. How can you tell? There are two simple ways – one is to notice whether your ankles become puffy especially towards the end of the day or after long periods of inactivity. If you press with your thumb on the inside of the calf just above the ankle and produce an indentation that does not disappear rapidly this is a sign of fluid retention. The second method is to press on the inside of your wrist, in the area of the crease between the hand and the wrist, and notice if a bubble appears within the crease. You need to practise this several times until you find the right spot – it is slightly on the 'hand' side of the crease. If a bubble appears – especially if it is large – this is another symptom that you are overloaded. How often you urinate is another symptom of excess fluid intake. Chinese called urine the new gold and the bowel movement the old gold. If our condition is more yin urination is frequent, the colour of water and likely to have little or no odour. When our condition becomes tight, concentrated or yang the urine becomes less, is darker and smells strongly.

One of the problems of being overloaded with fluid is that liquid itself is heavy. Consequently too much fluid will make us feel heavy, tired and lethargic. The kidneys, whose function it is to filter this fluid on an hourly basis, are often regarded in the West as filters and electrolyte balancers. We are advised to drink plenty of fluid to 'flush' them out. However, if you are tired, and you drink more, you are only giving the kidneys more work to do. It is wiser to find the right balance and not to overload the system.

Naturally when it is hot we are attracted to drinks that have a cooling effect – ice-cold liquids, tropical fruit juices and drinks that are high in sugar. All of these have a yinizing effect. Hot drinks, whether they be soups or simple teas, generally have a more 'warming' yang effect. On a cold, damp winter's morning when we feel unenthusiastic, probably the worst drink to have is a large glass of ice-cold orange juice. On the other hand, certain teas that are high in caffeine and certainly coffee have a very stimulating effect on the adrenal glands and the nervous system. But this sensation of 'yangization' can be misleading and false, really only a hollow and superficial effect. If you have ever been to a meeting where ideas and new projects are on the agenda and plenty of coffee is consumed, then the ideas roll. However, in my experience, they often lack roots or sufficient grounding. I think of a meeting that is driven by coffee as something like a car leaving the traffic lights, making a lot of noise and creating an image of dynamic movement. It's just the wheels are spinning. In the end nothing is gained.

Water must be regarded as the essential form of liquid nutrient for the body. It is abundant in nature and clearly present within ourselves. The quality of this water is fundamentally behind the basis of our health. Good quality water is fresh, bright and well oxygenated. The best water to find is often impractical in terms of our current way of life but is ideally drawn from a spring. Early farms, settlements and villages were strategically placed so that they could benefit from a good source of water. The health and welfare of the entire community was essentially founded on the water 'source'. It is interesting to note that 60 per cent of the world's surface is covered by liquid, that 60 per cent of our own body's volume is liquid and that 60 per cent of the world's diseases are also water borne. Water is a fundamental quality of our human life.

Nowadays our choice of water is limited to bottled spring water, filtered metropolitan water or unfiltered metropolitan water. Of these three choices then the best would be fresh local spring water if it is available. In traditional times we drew water from our local well or spring and in the same way nowadays we need to have a source of water that is as close as possible. Rather than being persuaded to buy foreign or exotic bottled spring water, find a source that originates near your home. Then the water has come from the same environment that you are living in. It is still not as ideal as getting the water direct from the spring as even bottle spring water can be months old – and time diminishes the quality of Chi that water has within it. Although filtering our water supply can take away many undesirable elements, it does leave a product that is a little too 'sanitized'. Water is not only H_2O but a number of other elements that, in their own way, supply variety and freshness to our system. Filtering metropolitan water makes the product cleaner but equally renders it almost sterile.

The worst form of water for us to use is undoubtedly metropolitan water straight from the tap. In some cities this water has been recycled some seven or eight times. During the process it loses its Chi and essential vitality. If we drink this water all the time, it is only when we go away from its source and taste something different that we realize how sterile and tasteless that water is. We can all recall at some point in our lives drinking straight from a mountain stream and noticing not only its freshness and its taste but the sheer joy of its Chi. It is this quality that is difficult to either bottle or quantify.

Another form of liquid intake in our culture is alcohol. Different cultures create different forms of this by either fermentation or distillation. Local grains or fruits are used in the process and historically traditional people would use alcohol for celebration and other social gatherings. While it is recognized that consuming alcohol is intoxicating, it is important to remember that it is also a depressant (yinizing). Although initially warming the next step is that alcohol calms and relaxes you. Much of its effect depends on our own condition and, to some degree, our constitution. Individuals whose condition is relatively yin need only a small amount of this concentrated form of yin to feel the effect very quickly. On the contrary, people who are excessively yang seem to manage to consume greater amounts of alcohol before it affects their condition. Popular current medical theory argues that a small amount of beer or wine daily can prevent the risk of coronary heart disease. Since a heart attack is essentially an excessive yang manifestation, a small amount of relaxing yin could arguably offset this imbalance. Perhaps there are other yin foods or drinks that could do the same job. The effects of yin in alcohol brings out different emotional expressions in people, depending on their current condition. These can range from being garrulous, insensitive, aggressive, uninhibited to depressed. Governments and medical experts are constantly advising us on 'safe' levels of alcohol consumption for adult males and females. This is measured purely statistically and scientifically. If you do drink regularly and 'feel the need' to have a drink to relax or to forget then it would be wise to take stock of this during the 10-day re-balance programme. Here are a few useful pointers and questions that can act as guidelines in helping you to determine whether your consumption of alcohol has become excessive for your current condition.

- Does your mood swing quickly after having a drink?
- Are you finding yourself more dependent on a drink?

- Do you rely on alcohol to 'unwind' you at the end of the day?
- Do you rely on alcohol to give you confidence?
- Are you more likely to have a drink when you feel depressed or despondent?
- Do you become increasingly arrogant, obsessive, aggressive or insensitive when you have a drink?
- Are you failing to keep your promises and commitments?
- Are you starting to avoid family and close friends who may call you to task over your drinking?
- If you do drink regularly and fairly heavily – are there signs that it is affecting your physical condition? For example, do you feel more tired and are you looking older?

If you recognize that your behaviour patterns follow several of these points on an increasingly regular basis, and if deep down you realize that you have a problem, then indeed you have. It is best to seek professional help or counselling before you spiral into a downward path of chronic alcohol dependency.

The effect of food

As you will have discovered from the beginning of this section, food is the least important of these four factors in terms of our day-to-day survival. However, unlike Chi, air or liquid, where we have limited control over the quality and quantity of what we absorb, we have full control over most of what we eat. It is up to us to select, prepare and eat our food. A chocolate bar does not fly out of a confectioner's shop, unwrap itself and disappear down our throats! We have the freedom to buy it or not. One of the secrets to understanding the importance of food to our condition is to realize that as human beings we have evolved over many thousands of years. Part of our evolution has been dependent on what we ate. Rather like a fuel-efficient engine of the future we need to consider our 'fuel' in relation to our needs and see that any 'waste products' are eliminated easily without running the risk of clogging up the system. In other words, if we can design a diet that efficiently uses food without causing a build-up of excess within the system, then we are on the road toward enjoying a healthy body which in turn is a vehicle for an adventurous and creative life. As the Yellow Emperor reveals in the *Nei Ching*, we should aim to eat and live in harmony with the seasons, our activity and our condition. Here now are the principles of yin and yang applied to food, the conclusions of which you can see in Section Two (p. 139) when you design the dietary part of your 10-day programme.

The ingredients

All food will have components of yin and yang within them – expansion/concentration, sweetness/savoury, soft/hard, vegetable/animal, summer or winter grown. If we begin with the yin end of the spectrum the foods that fall into this category are: sugar, spice, alcohol, tropical fruits, fruit juices, peppers, tomatoes, salads, milk, yoghurt and oil. Foods at the yang end include: salt, soya sauce, eggs, meat, poultry, paté, smoked fish, toast, crackers, savoury snacks. The middle of the spectrum, with fair amounts of both yin and yang qualities, include: cereal grains, vegetables, salads, pulses, white meat, fish, seeds, nuts, cheese, temperature climate foods, bread and pasta.

However, this simple view of the food spectrum sees them only for the raw and Chi value that they hold.

Cooking styles

In the hustle and bustle of modern life few of us have the time to prepare intricately balanced meals that involve several cooking styles and many different ingredients. However, the principles of traditional oriental cooking are invaluable, and I am deeply grateful for this early discipline that I studied – and still practise today in a more liberal form.

The more yang forms of cooking apply more time to the cooking process, use a higher flame, cook with some form of pressure – be it a pressure cooker or an oven – and finally use salt or its by-products in the cooking process. The higher the content of any of these factors makes the food more yang. Conversely, the less time a dish takes to prepare – like a salad or blanching vegetables quickly – the more the food is prepared in a yin fashion. The use of little or no flame in cooking, minimal or no use of salt and finally the lack of 'pressure' in the preparation all endow the ingredients with a higher degree of yin.

If we look at the spectrum of cooking styles from yin to yang the sequence would be: raw, marinated, steamed, boiled, short sauté, long sauté, deep fry, bake and roast.

Making the balance

When you allow your current condition to dictate what you eat and how you prepare it, you are likely to end up with more of the same. When you feel cold, damp, tired and unenthusiastic you are far more likely to reach for a soggy salad, a limp sandwich or a meal that requires very little preparation. However, a warm-hearted, hot, rich meal would re-invigorate you. When you are too yang, uptight, busy and hyperactive – you are more likely to choose food which matches this condition. This could include pizza, a hamburger, deep fried fish and chips – some kind of food that is very hot, salty or savoury that will give you even more heat and energy. It is therefore essential that we take into account our current condition before we select the ingredients for our meal and decide upon a cooking style that would benefit us. For example, if you came home one evening feeling particularly 'yang' and the only food you had available was salmon – which is also a relatively yang food – you would be wise to prepare it to balance your condition, in the least yang style. You could eat it raw or marinated, steamed or poached. You would be wise to avoid baking or deep frying it as this would only make you more yang.

Another consideration regarding your ingredients and cooking styles is the season of the year. Generally in the warmer and hotter months, which are yang, you need more cooling and relaxing foods, especially from the vegetable kingdom. Minimize your intake of salty, heavy animal foods and fats. However, in the colder, damper winter months we all benefit from food that has been prepared with more fire, time, pressure and salt – soups, stews and casseroles – even our desserts at this time of the year can be warm and well cooked.

The third area to consider in relation to choosing foods that are appropriate to ourselves is the kind of activity we are engaged in. When I was nineteen years old, I put in 14-hour shifts, 13 days a fortnight for 4 months in a mine in the Northern Territory of Australia. Before going down the shaft at 7 a.m. we all ate like kings: eggs, bacon, chops, even steaks. We had plenty of bread and sautéed potatoes, delicious fruits and all the varieties of cereals available. We all loaded as if this were our last meal! During the shift underground we had a bag of sandwiches to last the day and when we returned to the surface at around 9 p.m. the canteen was closed and most of us would fall into bed exhausted and uninterested in eating anyway. When you eat such high protein foods with enormous calorific value it is essential that you use it. Where otherwise does all the excess energy go? Certainly it does not improve your artistic or creative skills but needs to be burnt off physically. If we are incapable of doing this the excess will form itself into fat and burden us in turn in so many ways.

I became a vegetarian in 1976 and made this choice purely because I was suspicious about the quality of meat that was available when I began to live in England. Compared to meat that I had bought in markets throughout the world it looked and tasted 'artificial'. I even gave up fish and all dairy products. But although I changed the ingredients I had not yet mastered the principles of yin and yang cooking styles. It was a hot summer that year and I was living on basically vegetable food, mainly raw, but my job was a packer in a deep freeze for a large ice-cream manufacturer. With the very hot summer there was an increased demand for ice-cream and the pay was very good. At the beginning of the shift we dressed up like Eskimos; yet despite all the protective layers I felt very, very cold. During the breaks it took me far longer than my colleagues to get warm. I would sit shivering in the sunshine for half an hour at lunch time and would dread having to go back into the deep freeze. I was far too yin! I was rescued a few weeks later by a martial arts instructor who made the simple suggestion, 'Why don't you put some fire into your food?' It is in extreme situations that we begin to see new perspectives. For me this experience proved to be a turning point and it led me to study and practise what is essentially an age-old alchemical process – balancing our food and cooking styles with our condition, the seasons and our activity.

Conclusion

Our constitution, which we are born with, is unlikely to change and reveals our potential and capacity in life. However, our condition is in a constant state of change and it is dependent on the four factors of Chi, air, water and food for how it manifests. Given that you have some choice in the matter, you can work on many of these factors relative to your condition to enjoy greater health and the consequent freedom that this brings.

4

Oriental Diagnosis: Self-Assessment

'Self-examination, if it is thorough enough, is nearly always the first step toward change. I was to discover that no one who learns to know himself remains just what he was before.'

Thomas Mann

The purpose of this chapter is to help you assess your current condition so that you can, in Section Two, design your own unique 10-day re-balance programme. The unique feature of this style of self-assessment is that it allows you to see yourself from many different perspectives. Your current condition is primarily based on the four major influences that were outlined in Chapter 3 – food, liquid, oxygen and Chi. In this chapter instead of having, for example, your blood examined, or your iris, or completing a stress questionnaire, you will be able to cover many aspects of your physical and emotional well-being with the techniques provided.

It is vital to remember that, unlike our constitution, our condition is constantly changing. Therefore, in terms of your condition, who you discover you are today is not necessarily true of who you were yesterday or who you will be next week. So do not label yourself as yin or yang or as having a weak liver! That is merely something that may show up today.

HOW DOES IT WORK?

Diagnosing yourself is far more of a challenge than having someone else assess your condition. The reason is that you see yourself through your own condition. If you feel tired then you are likely to see the world through tired eyes. If you are impatient and irritable your experience of the world around you will be coloured by your own feeling of impatience and irritability. As George Bernard Shaw wrote in *Man and Superman*: 'Better keep yourself clean and bright: you are the window through which you must see the world.'

All of us have the capacity to diagnose using the methods that will be outlined later in this chapter. They are primarily based on our senses, in particular our intuition, by which we naturally pick up a lot of information. Using this basic capacity for assessing Chi energy, oriental diagnosis takes the process further.

Some methods of oriental diagnosis do not lend themselves easily to self-assessment. There is obviously no 'polarity' between yourself and yourself. However, the methods which we will cover are fine for assessing your current condition, and remember that it is the overall flavour of a preponderance towards yin or yang that you need to pick up on to form an opinion or conclusion.

Oriental diagnosis is primarily based on our senses. These include touch, hearing, smelling, seeing and sensing. Practitioners are encouraged to begin their assessment from the 'big picture'. This means that they are unlikely to begin a diagnosis by feeling the pulses, which are very detailed, but rather by sensing or feeling how a person appears to them. Another way of expressing this argument is to start with the big picture (yin) and head down the list of different techniques towards the details (yang).

Diagnosis by sensing

To do this well you need the greatest possible polarity with, or distance from the person you are observing. That is why when you meet someone for the first time you can sense immediately how they are feeling. As you interact and communicate with them more, that capacity diminishes. Whenever one of my children has been ill, I have always found it very difficult to assess or pick up on what is going on intuitively, while a colleague or another parent who has that polarity, rarely has difficulty in sensing what may be wrong.

Diagnosis by odour

Our skin, our breath, our stools and our urine all carry an odour which is indicative of what we are currently eliminating. Naturally, one way to monitor our current condition is to be aware of what we are 'discharging'. Any deficiency or excess of toxins within the body will show up not only in terms of how we feel but also in how we 'smell'. Rather like the previous method of diagnosis (by senses) you do not have the polarity with yourself to benefit greatly from this method. However, unusually strong odours that emanate from the stools or the urine are a reflection that your condition is too yang. Some of these smells can be described as putrid, burnt, rancid, foul or sweet.

Little or no odour is an indication of a yin condition.

You may recall at some time in your life visiting a friend or relative who had been in bed for a day or two with a bad cold or fever and, on entering the room, noticing a strong smell in the atmosphere. An experienced practitioner of oriental diagnosis can ascertain very quickly from the particular odour whether a person's condition is more yin or more yang and even which organ is involved. Being able to eliminate or discharge is a healthy function of the body, and the symptoms, such as the odour, are indicative of what is being eliminated and which organ is involved.

Diagnosis by listening

Have you noticed that your voice, rather like your handwriting, changes regularly? Both are indications of your current condition. The first time you pick up your pen to write a note in the morning you may notice whether your stroke is firm, direct and clear (yang) or spidery, weak and loosely composed (yin). In the same way your voice expresses in terms of yin or yang how your condition is today. It is revealed in the intonation of the voice, its power and clarity. Whether it is the first greeting you make, the opening sentences in a business meeting or your first telephone conversation – your tone is an indication to you and, on a subtle level, to whoever you are communicating with as to how you feel today.

If our current condition is more yin, caused by either a lack of yangizing factors in our lifestyle or by the consumption of excess yin – wine, sugar, coffee, etc. – then our voice comes across on a higher pitch than usual. Yin also shows up in speaking more slowly with a dampness or wetness to the voice. This can sound as if we are on the edge of tears. The voice can also appear feeble, soft and even shaky. A tendency to be quieter than usual is also considered a sign of being more yin.

When our overall condition is currently more yin we feel more vulnerable than usual. This will lead to self-protection and defensiveness which itself leads to many of the qualities of expression that are listed above. Try listening to the message that you leave on the answerphone and see if you were more yin or more yang when you made the recording.

The more yang quality of voice is deeper or dry and frequently faster. When we are hyperactive we talk quicker, and when we are experiencing a deep fever (yang) there is often a point when we become extremely garrulous, making little or no sense to those around us. Our voice can come across as impatient and pushy; we are very direct and frequently loud in our communication.

Remember that your condition is changing from day to day

and next time you are in a conversation or a meeting, be aware of how your voice comes across and for practice listen to the expression of others around you. It will give you more insight into this level of diagnosis. It is also particularly helpful when you listen to a friend or relative on the telephone. They may be telling you some story regarding a relationship or situation at work, but at the same time they are conveying another story in terms of their expression. Does their voice come across as over yang – very hyper, talkative, loud and pushy? Do they seem more vulnerable and yang when their expression is slower, softer, slightly feeble and withdrawn?

Diagnosis by seeing

This is a relatively easy way of assessing your condition on a yin/yang basis. Remember, as a guideline in diagnosis start from the biggest possible view. This means that you need to look at yourself initially from the big perspective and then narrow down your observations towards the details.

Vitality

To pick up on this area of your health, you need to take a quick glance at yourself in the mirror. Not a long protracted stare! Just a quick glance will reveal your level of vitality. The area where this shows up the most clearly is the eyes. A quick glance reveals your level of vitality at the moment. Tired and dull eyes indicate a currently yin condition whereas bright sharp eyes indicate a more yang condition.

Body language

How you move your body, your walk, your gait and how you sit can all reveal your current state of well-being. The faster and more direct your way of walking, the more yang your condition. A slow, ponderous and meandering approach indicates a more yin condition. On your way to work you can be aware of your condition while travelling on public transport, tackling an escalator or walking along the pavement. Are you cautious? Do you give way to others? Do you indicate to people approaching you that you are not clear whether you are going to the left or right? These are yin expressions of your condition. If you have a tendency to make a bee-line to your destination, to trot up the escalators or show no hesitancy to other pedestrians – then your condition is more yang.

If in a meeting or conversation your body appears relaxed, calm and centred then your condition leans towards yang. If you punctuate your expression with your hands and keep both feet on the floor, your current condition is more yang. If, however, your shoulders are more stooped and you have a tendency to cross your arms across either your chest or your abdomen and feel more comfortable with your legs cross then these indications of self-protection are a current sign of a generally more yin condition.

Several years ago I watched an American documentary in which they interviewed young muggers. After initially asking them why and how they got involved in this sort of crime the presenter showed them footage of pedestrians walking along a pavement. They were asked to pick out potential targets for mugging. Without any collusion with one another they all picked the same individuals which, from a diagnostic and body language perspective, all bore the same hallmarks – they were more yin, vulnerable. Later in the programme the youngsters were also asked to pick out individuals that they would not mug. Here again they were unanimous about whom they would avoid. They had chosen to avoid those individuals that had a more yang approach in their body language and walking style.

The skin

We can take a lot of time cleaning, preparing and observing our skin. Since it is regarded in the Orient as an elimination system, then the symptoms that can manifest in the skin are a good indication of our current condition. To begin with, if our skin is dull or slightly bloated our condition is more yin. Press with your thumb into the skin and see how quickly the dimple that the pressure forms reverts to a natural level. The slower this return to normal the more yin your condition. Very dry skin can often be a sign of an over yang condition whereas bright and shiny skin is a sign of balance and harmony. In oriental medicine, the skin can be regarded as the third lung or third kidney. The quality of our skin and its inherent health is based on our internal condition. Diet, oxygen, fluid and environmental factors play the biggest role in the creation of healthy skin, together with the capacity of the internal elimination organs to function well. In the modern world, however, there is a tendency to approach skin care from a completely opposite perspective. Most skin treatments are designed to be applied on to the surface and whether these are cleansing agents or moisturizers, they are simply dealing with the skin condition symptomatically and not taking into account some of the fundamental causes of the skin's health.

The meridians

A huge area of oriental diagnosis is centred on the study of the channels of Chi energy that pass across the surface of the body along pathways known as meridians. There are fourteen of these channels on the surface of the body and they connect with the internal organs, their partners and the systems that co-ordinate breathing, circulation and elimination. The concept of Chi and the meridians is fundamental to oriental medicine. For the purpose of this book you do not need to study fourteen meridians and approximately 370 points. However, unusual symptoms, rashes, tingling and aches can be correlated to individual meridians. The Chi energy in meridians flows like water in a river. It has the potential to be erratic and gushing and bubbling like a mountain stream or slow and ponderous like a river on the

A simple map of the meridians

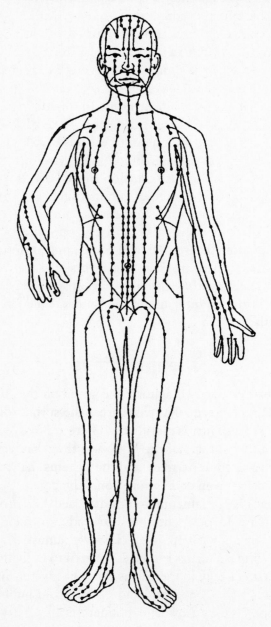

lowland plains, and can take on the quality of stagnant water in an old pond or even a rusty tin can at the bottom of a garden.

To use this approach to diagnosis as to whether your condition is more yin or yang, begin to notice when unusual symptoms appear either on the surface or just below. If you can identify any of the symptoms listed below in the yin or yang categories, check them against the chart above to see which meridian and hence organ is involved:

Yin:	Yang:
flaccid muscles	stiff or tight muscles
dull aches	sharp pain
cold sensations	hot or tingly sensations
white, pale or greenish tinge to skin	rashes or spots that feel hot or irritable or have a stronger red or purple colour within them

Hair

In much the same way as you might check the coat of your dog or cat to assess the animal's health, hair is a very good indication of well-being. Although its deeper qualities reflect our overall nutritional balance, its changing day-to-day quality is very much an indication of our current health. Tired hair has a direct correlation with tiredness in us – a yin condition. Bouncy bright hair represents yang vitality. Other indications are:

Yin	Yang
losing hair	curly hair
damp or greasy hair	dry hair
hair which lacks 'sparkle'	brittle hair

The length of our hair can also influence our condition. For example, having our hair cropped short is a yangizing process. Cutting back the hair is rather similar to pruning a plant. It allows new growth and new vitality to come through. The shorter the haircut – right down to completely shaving the head, the more yangizing the process is. Think of the imagery that very short hair creates. It can make an individual look more aggressive, more sharp, more bold or more 'male'. In its extreme, very long hair can have both a yin appearance and a yinizing effect. Extremely long hair brings with it an impression of softness, gentleness, femininity and flexibility.

The face

Our face can reveal not only our current condition but, on closer observation, which specific element and related organ is involved. By glancing in the mirror it is easy to determine whether your current complexion is either dark or very pale. Both of these are usually consistent with a yin, stagnant condition. But if our face is flushed with plenty of red or purple that is a clear sign of excess yang within the system. For example, if we are ill in bed or if we spend the weekend indoors with no fresh air or exercise our complexion can become pale or even dark. Take a rapid run around the block and come home breathless and sweaty and you will be flushed by the increased circulation which brings strong red or purple colour to your face.

In the very early stages of embryonic development, our body appears as one unit. However, during the first eighteen days or so a change occurs whereby what will later become our head begins to separate from the lower part which will become our body. As these two areas separate, there a connection remains that will continue throughout our development in embryo and into our adult lives. The reason is that our face has separated out of the areas that became our body where our internal organs are stored. By understanding this, it is easier to see why the following five areas of the face correlate to the five major internal organs.

Face Diagnosis

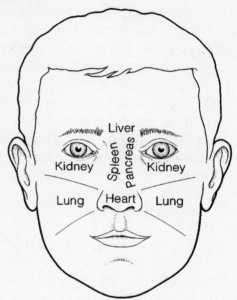

The lungs

We have two lungs and two cheeks, naturally left cheek and left lung correlate and vice versa. The upper section of our cheek relates to the upper part of our lung and the lower part of the cheek to the lower part of the lung. Looking in the mirror, check on the complexion of your cheeks – are they a good bright colour or are they sunken and pale (yin) or more puffy with many broken red capillaries (yang)? Small creamy spots that appear within the area of the cheeks can also be an indication of excess mucus currently lodged in the lungs. Good advice if this is the case, is to reduce or avoid mucus-forming food such as dairy products and raw fruit during this 10-day breakthrough programme.

The kidneys

The facial area that corresponds to the kidneys can be found just below the eyes. If this area appears watery, puffy, swollen or slightly red, it is an indication of a more yin – expansive – quality within the kidneys. This can be caused by excess fluid in the system or general tiredness with the resultant incapacity of kidney energy to work as hard as it could. If the area below the eyes appears dark, giving the impression of a bruise, then your condition is too 'tight' (yang). What is a bruise? Essentially this is where blood has become stuck, unable to flow or 'dammed up'. This bruised appearance below the eyes shows that the kidneys are tired and stagnant due perhaps to an excess of salt or not enough sleep or too much drain on the adrenal glands which are closely associated with the kidneys. Stress, not enough sleep and too much sexual activity can drain the adrenal glands.

The liver

Signs of imbalance within the liver can be found in the area between the eyebrows. A red or purple colour similar to an inflammation in this area is a sign of a more yin condition within the liver. This can be caused by too much alcohol, too much sugar, spices or the use of drugs. Deep or superficial lines in this area, either vertical or horizontal, indicate that the problem is more deep, therefore more yang. Overeating, late night eating and too much saturated animal fat are often the cause.

The heart

We have one heart and one nose – both are centrally located within the body or the face. When the tip of the nose becomes red or purple or, in more chronic situations, swollen, this is the sign that the heart energy has become more yin. This yin quality can manifest as 'swollen'. Excess fluids or excess fluid-based yin like fruit, fruit juice or alcohol could be a casual factor. When the tip of the nose appears white and pinched, a little like a white knuckle when you clench your fist, your condition has become too tight. This can be caused by too much salt but equally by being unable to release yang from the system, primarily stress. It is very important for the heart that we can release pent-up emotions and stress through activity and expression.

Pancreas and spleen

These are two very deep and central organs whose condition can show up on the bridge of the nose. Broken veins and capillaries on the surface of the bridge indicate a more yin condition as can a mild reddish or purple tinge to the skin. This can be caused by excess sugar in the system. A 'white knuckle' appearance shows a strong yang condition which, given that the pancreas is itself a very deep, active and yang organ, may well be a reaction to pre-dominantly yang excess. In terms of food these can include too much egg or hidden egg in cakes and biscuits, and hard dairy products such as cheese.

Have a glance in the mirror to see if you can determine a) whether you are yin or yang today, or b) if you can pick up which of the organs may be involved. Please do not become neurotic about this; remember that it is only one facet of diagnosis and, although our condition is constantly altering, the reactions that I have described above are perhaps the slowest to change.

The eyes

Traditional people have always regarded the eyes as the window into the soul or spirit, that intangible quality of energy which could equally be described as Chi and is primarily a yin mani-festation. A more yang description which the eyes can also represent is their relation to our nervous system. A very high percentage of what we perceive in the outside world is brought to us through the eyes – as is the high proportion of oriental diagnosis that is based on seeing or observation. A simple expression of our nervous system would be to divide it into a) the capacity to receive information and b) the capacity to respond accordingly. When our overall nervous system becomes excessively yin or excessively yang this will affect not only what we perceive but how we react as well.

When our nervous system becomes more yin our perception can be slower and our consequent reaction equally slow. We can dither, we can procrastinate, we can be unclear about what we are trying to achieve. When our nervous system is more yang our perception and reaction is very clear, quick and precise. How do we assess this in terms of our current condition?

Signs that your nervous system may currently be more yin are: if your eyes have a tendency to 'drift' when you are in conversation. You avoid looking directly in the eyes of the person speaking to you. Or you blink frequently. Normally we blink approximately three times a minute; more than this and the nervous system is currently more yin.

Signs that your nervous system is very yang at present include: the capacity to 'lock on' to someone else's gaze; to blink less than three times a minute; a tendency to 'tunnel vision' when it comes to conversations or while attempting to discuss the broader

San Paku

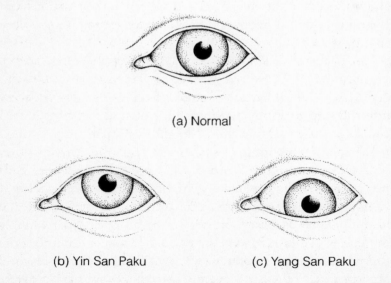

(a) Normal

(b) Yin San Paku   (c) Yang San Paku

issues of a subject. Poor (yin) or sharp (yang) hand/eye co-ordination are another very good indication of the nervous system's current state.

In Japan they have a very interesting system of diagnosis based purely on observing the position of the eye within its socket.

In the diagram opposite, example a) shows a normal eye. That is, the top and bottom of the iris touch the upper and lower eye-lid and two clear whites of the eye are visible either side of the iris. Example b) shows what the Japanese called yin san paku. This is where a third area of white is visible below the eye. The transla-tion of san paku from the Japanese is three (*san*) whites (*paku*). This upward tilting of the eye is regarded as a sign of vulnerabil-ity. Being vulnerable is a yin condition which means that we are potentially 'off guard'. In Japan, people with this condition were thought to be vulnerable to ill health, theft, robbery, accident or becoming the victim of a situation. An individual who is yin san paku could be the victim of loss of money in an investment or loss of position or job through poor judgement or intuition.

In example c) a third white appears but this time above the eye. This condition is known as yang san paku. Here the indi-vidual appears to be looking down slightly. When the nervous system has become too yang the individual is likely to be sensi-tive to the outside world and may cause trouble to others, often unconsciously, by a stubborn or inflexible approach to whatever they are doing. These people have the potential to cause acci-dents, become violent or manic. If you get into a heated discus-sion with someone and it leads to an argument, watch their eyes! If they become yang san paku, back off!

When eyes tile either upwards or downwards, as in examples b) and c), then naturally the world appears 'off centre'. This means that our judgement and our perception of about what is going on is equally off centre. The yin san paku can make us the victim whereas the yang san paku is far more likely to make us the insensitive causal factor of trouble. Towards the end of life and close of death, human beings' eyes begin to display signs of yin san paku, and upon death, the eyes slowly roll upwards.

Death is the ultimate yin state. At the other end of the life's spectrum, when we are born, our eyes are yang san paku. Next time you see a new born baby notice that, firstly, they hardly ever blink, and secondly, they have yang san paku.

Our eyes also reveal our overall vitality. This quality can also be described as our current Chi. When our eyes appear tired, dull or lifeless our condition is too yin. When our eyes appear bright and sparkling our condition is much more yang. If you have ever been to buy fresh fish in a market located near the sea, you will know that one of the most tried and tested methods of assessing whether the fish is fresh is to examine the eyes. Naturally, bright sparkling eyes show a fresh fish whereas dull, glazed or opaque eyes indicate a fish that is past its sell-by date. Diagnosing other peoples' eyes is something that we do unconsciously all our lives: when we meet someone, when we are in a meeting; and it is the key to success in any martial art.

Touch

A very simple method of assessing your current condition is by checking whether the palms of your hands are cold/hot, damp/dry. To do this effectively, lightly pass the back of one of your hands over the surface of the other palm. Repeat this several times until you have a true sense. Damp and cold are yin – dry and hot are yang.

Whenever we shake hands with someone this exchange is a diagnostic technique. While we feel the vitality (Chi) in their grip we inevitably look them in the eye and ask 'How do you do?' or 'How are you?' The firmer their grip the more yang they are – a damp, soft handshake reveals a more yin condition.

How firm is your grip at the moment? Do the muscles and tendons in your fingers, hand and wrist appear firm or are they loose? The strength of your grip does vary from day to day, as you may have discovered when trying to open a tight lid on a jar or bottle. Some days it is easy, some days you have to ask a neighbour.

Next you can check how firm or flaccid the flesh is on the inside of your wrist. If you apply pressure to this area with your thumb does it create an indentation which takes time to revert to normal or does it bounce back immediately? The sign of a healthy condition is that the flesh reverts to its normal level very quickly. If your condition is more yin a dimple will form which could take anything up to 15 seconds to revert, whereas with an excessively yang condition the flesh will hardly give and there is a lot of resistance to any pressure. This is a common method for diagnosing fresh fish at the market – apply some pressure to the flesh and see whether the dimple you form reverts fairly quickly. Stale or stagnant fish will remain 'bruised'.

If you are very sensitive to the touch and have a tendency to bruise easily then your condition is more yin, while people who are not ticklish and are insensitive to pressure or pain are much more yang. Therefore, when someone with a yang nature (constitution) and a yang condition complains of pain, he or she really is in pain!

Acupoints along the meridians of the body can also provide useful diagnostic pressure points for you to try. It is a huge area of study and practise but should you find a point that is painful but with a dull sensation this is an indication of yin. Sharp, tingly sensations upon pressure are usually a good indication of yang stagnation.

The pulse

The most yang, the most accurate and the most up-to-date of all the diagnostic techniques is the study of the pulses. Clinical oriental medicine regards this as the foundation stone of their diagnostic techniques. Pulse diagnosis gives a very complete and accurate up-to-the-minute assessment of your condition.

The imagery that the pulse invokes is that of the rhythm of a river, and the language used in traditional Chinese medicine is all connected with descriptions of different states of water as it travels. There are twelve pulses in the body which connect to the major organs and eighteen different interpretations which can be multiplied by these twelve. It is a huge study but we will look only at one of the more practical uses here to help you assess whether you are more yin or yang at the time.

The best way to locate a pulse for this exercise is to find the small protrusion on the inside of your wrist on the same side as the thumb. Bring your opposite hand across and place the palm of your hand over the back of the wrist, curling your middle finger round over the bony protrusion to find the hollow beyond. Gently feel around until you find a pulse. The best time of day to check your pulse is when you wake and leave the yin state of sleep to enter the yang phase of activity. While in this semi-restful state you will get a more accurate picture than if you were to take your pulse at midday having run up three flights of stairs. A normal pulse will beat four times during the entire inhalation and exhalation process. It will appear soft and regular. When our condition is more yin the pulse will be slower than this, feel very soft, thin, thready and weak. A pulse that indicates a more yang condition will be faster, throbbing, pushing and present the image of flooding.

I had this method of diagnosis tried out on me in 1972 while crossing the border from Afghanistan into Iran. All the Europeans that were entering Iran were taken into a large open customs shed and politely invited to put their suitcases on a bench for inspection. The customs officer questioning me kept a firm fix on my eyes with his, and while his left hand was attached to my wrist observing my pulse his right hand was rummaging in my suitcase. It was certainly a bright idea but a formidable experience! My pulse was like a Geiger counter as his hand searched. When I passed the initial test he applied the same practice to a body search. It was a very unnerving experience but it proved accurate in the ensuing minutes. While I was repacking my bag the same officer using the same methods managed to find a large quantity of drugs hidden in the clothing of the next person. No X-ray machines, no specially trained dogs just pulse diagnosis did the job.

Diagnosis by questioning

In the final method of diagnosis you can begin to assess your current condition by being aware of any symptoms and habits you may have. Unfortunately it is much easier for a third party to see these traits and to draw some form of diagnosis from them as you are in a sense too close to the situation. So far as symptoms are concerned, begin to notice whether aches and pains have a dullness about them or appear gradually and fade gradually (yin). Symptoms that come on fast and can equally disappear fast but have a sharp, acute nature are more yang.

If symptoms appear at night or we have difficulty sleeping at night or prefer to be more active at night, our condition is more yin. If symptoms have a tendency to appear during the day or we have a preference for small amounts of sleep at night and have difficulty slowing down and resting our condition is more yang.

How do you go about things on a day-to-day basis? Are you scatty, do you chop and change your mind; are you slow? These are all yin qualities. If you are very fast, focused, unadaptable, rigid and pushy by nature your condition is more yang.

Conclusion

Armed with these new insights based on oriental diagnosis you will be able to determine whether your current condition is more yin or more yang in Part Two. It is important to remember that you do not base your assessment purely on one model of diagnosis. It is far more accurate to go through the checklist there and to notice the tendency in your answers. This will lead you towards deciding whether you are currently more yin or more yang.

Remember also that your condition is constantly changing. Whatever conclusion you come to in Part Two regarding your current condition, please avoid making the mistake of labelling yourself yin or yang for ever. Within a few hours, days or weeks it will be possible to change your condition into its opposite, either by slow gentle means or more 'violent' methods. If you were very yin you could jump straight into an icy cold bath and immediately become yang!

Practising many of the techniques outlined above is an excellent way to develop a skill in this area. Watching and listening to people around you in a non-judgemental way is the most practical way of taking the subject on. Diagnosis is a Greek word which literally means *dia* (through) *gnosis* (knowledge). Diagnosis is not just a clinical skill but an intuitive art that all of us are capable of benefitting from and have been using all our lives. The insights that you can gain from observing and listening to others have also a profound effect on your understanding of yourself. Another benefit is that this system can help you to understand what other people's needs are in your relationship with them. When you listen to a friend who pours out his or her problems you can have the additional tool of really hearing them in terms of their current condition. Is their behaviour and understanding of the problem based on a more yin or yang condition? Then in your support or response you can take a more appropriate line of action. If their condition is more yin and they appear to be victimized, martyred or uninspired to take a stand, your advice can be of a more yangizing nature. You can talk straight, get to the point or approach them in such a way that it brings them face to face with the issue in hand. If, on the other hand, your friend is manifesting all or many of the symptoms of a too yang condition, then think of a way to help them soften, relax or yinize their approach. Whether this is in the form of sympathy or creating an atmosphere that helps them to relax, it can add a new dimension to helping them resolve their current situation.

Finally, do not attempt to use these techniques as a kind of parlour game. Rather than share any new-found insights, encourage others to discover the information for themselves. As with most new ideas or studies that we take on, at the beginning we can be very keen but lack the practice. It is only when you have gained some personal insight or experience, using yin and yang, in understanding your health that you can begin to share your knowledge with others.

PART TWO

The Programme

5

Making Changes

Part One essentially covered the principles of how our bodies work and how we live in a world of change, which can be polarized into yin and yang – a useful shorthand for understanding the basic 'code' at the heart of all life.

The intention of Part Two is to provide you with an insight into where you are, what you would like to achieve and finally the steps to take to initiate this change. By combining this in Step Three with the appropriate plan, you have the opportunity to find yourself at the end of the 10-day period in a state of balance where your life will be greatly benefited from this newfound intuition and harmony. Ten days is by no means a large demand on our time and energy to make a shift. By the end of that period you should be in a very clear space – physically, mentally and spiritually – able to enjoy your recharged body and intuition. Building a future from a place where judgement is not clouded by pressure or obscured by the effects of a condition that is too yin or too yang is unique, but the possibility is available to you if you follow the 10-day plan.

The logic is very simple. If our overall condition, lifestyle and health is veering towards yin (tired, indifferent, withdrawn, cautious) then you need to bring about more yang quality changes in your life. If you identify your current situation as being too yang (stubborn, impatient, irritable, hyperactive, intolerant) then you need to steer yourself towards yin. The more extreme your symptoms in either of these conditions, the further you need to steer in the opposite direction in the 10-day period.

The idea that we can achieve perfect balance in our lives is essentially a myth. Look around in nature and it is obvious that we are living in a changing world. You and I are constantly changing too, but it is the degree by which we change that makes the difference. The more extreme our work, our diet, our lifestyle, the more demands made on us to bring about balance. It is the enormous swings that can leave us inefficient, tired, stressed and potentially unclear as to what we want. The turbulence of constant swings is a very inefficient use of our energy which ultimately can erode our health and our intuition. However, if we were by chance to find perfect balance (space), I am convinced that our lives would be very boring! There needs to be some form of dynamic, some kind of spark to give us creativity and a broad perspective on life.

The most common mistake in adopting the model of balance is to assume that we are always at the centre. The truth is that we are constantly shifting from yin to yang and vice versa. The further we swing in one direction the further we need to swing back in the other. But ideally we could be more effective, have more stamina and enjoy a wider perspective of ourselves and our future if our swings could be less violent and most centred on the fulcrum. When we identify that our condition is more yang, what we are really saying is that the fulcrum in this model of balance has shifted in the direction of yang (and the same for yin).

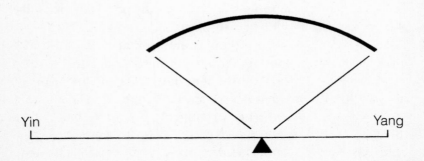

Yin   Yang

By the end of the ten-day period you will be passing through the central area, and that is the time to enjoy the benefits of this new-found perspective. However, there is a warning. If you follow the advice for too long you are likely to pass through this central balanced zone and begin to swing too far in the other direction. The ten-day programme provides you with the opportunity to be in this central zone at the *end* of the ten-day period. From within this space you will have a fresh new perspective in all areas of your life, and when you reintroduce old habits, you will have a clearer picture of how these factors affect your life. Take the plan to its extreme and swing too far the other way and you will lose the opportunity that this new perspective can offer. Remember also that if you discover that your current condition is strongly yang or yin you need to make an equally strong effort in the ten-day period to steer in the opposite direction. Small adjustments in your lifestyle are not likely to bring about any big shift.

STEP ONE – KNOWING WHO AND WHERE YOU ARE

This is an essential priority in undertaking any enterprise involving change. Knowing 'who' you are relates to understanding your unique constitution using oriental diagnosis. Knowing 'where' you are is being able to discern your current condition based not only on the oriental diagnosis that was covered in Chapter 4, but also how you are responding in terms of yin and yang to various areas in your life. These include your physical and recreational activities, what kinds of level of stress you have in your life and how you cope with them, your home and work environment, how you tackle issues in your life in relationship to old patterns of behaviour, diagnosis of your current energy/spirit and finally a current assessment of your diet.

Through the step by step self-assessment questionnaire in

Chapter 6 you will be able to conclude whether your overall current condition is leaning more towards yin or yang.

STEP TWO – PLANNING THE VOYAGE

Once you have established your current condition you need to be clear about what you would like to achieve. Here we look at the importance of the mind and how we can harness its power to achieve our goal. Through a guided visualization exercise you will be able to see yourself in the future and then design the practical steps it will take to reach that future. With these guidelines you will begin to live into that future. Unlike previous experiences of this kind of exercise, where you may have seen the possibility of a new future but listened to past negative experiences, this time you are encouraged to be in the present and to make that future present now!

STEP THREE – SETTING OFF

At this stage you have already identified, in Step One, who and where you are, you are clear about what you want to achieve from the visualization process in Step Two, and you need to identify the action to be taken through one of the two plans that you design for yourself in Step Three. One of the plans will have a more yangizing effect while the other will be more yinizing. Having already identified which direction you need to follow, you have six areas to work on:

- Activity
- Stress
- Environment
- Pattern/behaviour

- Spirit
- Diet

Within each of these areas are a number of practical suggestions for bringing change. Having assessed your current condition in Step One, you may feel, for example, that the current stagnation in your life relates to your lack of suitable physical activity or recreation. Perhaps your lifestyle is too sedentary and you need to choose an activity plan that has a 'yang' effect. Maybe your current diet is tipped too far in favour of 'yang' cooking styles and ingredients, and making a shift for ten days towards a lighter (more yin) style of cooking would be more appropriate for balance. Ideally, choose one or perhaps two areas to work on and do them well, rather than taking on all the areas and only managing to complete them superficially. Often, the most effective ones to work on are those you would find the most challenging!

DEALING WITH CHANGE

Perhaps one of the most amusing insights I had in recent years was a definition of lunacy. Forget the clinical version, try this one for size. 'Doing the same things again, but expecting a different outcome.' How often do we tackle the same issues, the same problems time and time again but with the same approach. It's a little bit like accidentally slamming your fingers in a door and then thinking to yourself that if you tried it again it wouldn't hurt this time! If on a superficial, mechanical level we can appreciate the lunacy of the idea, then why are we sometimes incapable of applying the same principle to greater issues in our life? We have plenty of evidence that this approach has not worked before. Are we going to allow the same illogical impression to get in the way this time as well. Here are some valuable guidelines that can help us deal with change and the challenges that can be involved.

Change can be challenging

It can be relatively easy to decide that something needs to change. However, when you are in the middle of the process, it can look pretty rough and untidy. It is one thing to have this wonderful vision of how it is going to be but quite another to endure the mayhem around you while you are introducing the change. We have all had experience of builders and decorators in our homes. Having decided on a new scheme or a new layout our heart and mind is set on what it is going to be like in ten days' time. However, it is all too easy to overlook what a potentially disruptive situation is going to occur while the dust and the debris fly. When you change your job, one of the key elements in the decision is the belief that it will be better. However, as you adopt the new work schedule, learn the new systems and adapt to the new team around you, it can be tiring and challenging. However, it is important not to lose sight of your vision. Deep down you know that in the long term it is all for the better.

On a biological level, our body represents how we have been living, eating and being in the previous months and years. On this physical level, you are 'constructed' from your past. When you step in the way and declare that things are going to change around here, the body does not fall into line overnight. It will constantly remind you of how you were, how you lived and what you craved and enjoyed. After the ten-day period your new-found direction will be matched by a more co-operative body as well.

Friends, relations and partners act in very much the same way. They really know you best from your past – whether that was twenty years or five minutes ago. They can feel threatened by your desire to change. Perhaps they feel more comfortable having you the way you were. If you shared with them your vision of a new you or a new direction that you are to undertake it will often not match up with the you that, from time to time, is struggling with the challenges of making changes in these first ten days. Keep on purpose, stay on track. It is worth it in the end.

When we approach change from a position of desperation, fear or pressure, driven by those three reasons there is little room for adaptability, creativity or flexibility. There is also a short-term 'band aid' approach to the programme, a lack of a long-term vision of the deeper potential of what change can bring about for us, and this is usually unproductive too.

In the final analysis it is really up to us to have the motivation to make changes in our lives. None of us responds well when we are told by others that we need to change. At best, we may reflect on other people's views and at worst we can stubbornly and stoically resist them and even go further than this by emphasizing the very qualities that are being criticized. A somewhat typical human rebellious nature! So although I believe that we can derive the greatest insights from other people, the motivation to bring about action or change is undoubtedly of our own making. The most positive and powerful time to introduce change is when you are ready. This way it will be natural and spontaneous and you will be completely responsible. Coming at change in a positive and up-beat frame of mind, together with telling those people close to you what you are up to for the ten days, really sets you off on a good course.

The need to be flexible

Whenever we take on something new it is wise to be flexible and adaptable in the initial stages. As with any new gadget, such as a computer, we are liable to make mistakes in the learning process. Rather than being defeated by these, regard them as essential prerequisites for learning. It will take time to get the hang of the new system and you are more likely to be mechanical rather than intuitive in your approach.

A major reason for abandoning any programme is associated with the distraction that previous commitments and arrangements can cause. You can still fit these in and remember that it is this quality of flexibility and adaptability that is the hallmark of success in making changes. But sometimes we use the excuse of existing commitments for either putting off change or abandoning it halfway. If you have decided to make dietary changes in the ten-day programme and midway through the process are invited out for dinner, what are you going to do? You could either turn down the invitation and tell your host that you are unable to come because you are on a special diet – this implies that their cooking is somehow 'wrong', that what you are doing is more important and, worse, if you are very direct in your communication they could feel rejected. The flexible approach is to say that you are delighted to accept the invitation, that you are halfway through a special programme and would appreciate some simple cooking. There is no need to elaborate or send them a menu by fax or a copy of this book! When we are open, flexible and grateful we frequently find exactly what we want on the table. It is when we forewarn our host exactly what we can or cannot eat that we are most likely to encounter the biggest difficulty. It is far better to enjoy your host's food cooked with love, warmth and the anticipation of a great dinner party with friends, than to eat food that they have prepared especially for you perhaps under pressure and for which they have little skill or intuitive feel.

You need time and space

Ideally, to get the most out of the programme, look for a 'window' in your diary of ten days. Perhaps take some home leave that you are due. Rushing anything, implementing changes superficially, and having a thousand and one distractions do not help.

Feeling worse before feeling better

Any programme of change can have very distinct healing qualities, whether these are physical, mental or spiritual. But in the initial stages there is a natural reaction to the process, the inevitable physical side-effects that can be associated with biological change. These can include tiredness, headaches, depression and irritability. Also, old patterns of behaviour can emerge, falling back on previous solutions to problems or ways of being.

From an oriental perspective it can be appreciated that our body maintains its balance by eliminating what we do not need. A healthy day-to-day example of this process is through our urination, our bowel movement and our breathing. However, when we take on board more than we can cope with or if we introduce 'agents of change', then these normal routes of elimination can become more active, more acute and very sensitive. The kinds of symptoms that can occur include: digestive ups and downs – wind, loose bowels or constipation; frequent urination; excessive sweating; a chill or a fever; a cold; a cough. Feelings of: self-pity, cynicism, depression, anxiety, fear, irritability, hypersensitivity, hyperactivity or hysteria. Your skin may appear to be different – rashes, spots or a strong odour.

Many people do not experience any of these symptoms but several do. None of them are life threatening and, if viewed as a side-effect, they can be ridden out rather than being suppressed or neutralized. It has been my experience that the more physically active we are, the quicker and deeper the changes occur on a biological level and the more likely you are to experience one or more of the symptoms listed above. But remember that all these are healthy signs of elimination provided they do not last longer than a few days.

Commitment

It is important to stick to your chosen programme as closely as you can. Supposing, for example, you decide it would make a difference to your future well-being if you took fifteen minutes to meditate every afternoon. Perhaps you had decided to do this because you had found that this was the most stressful part of your day. You make a commitment that you will do this for ten days knowing that it will rub off on your being and that after the ten days you will be feeling a lot more relaxed. You will have made a shift. However, miss a few sessions during the ten days or, worse, substitute your 15 minutes of relaxation with a heated argument and you are beginning to revert to your old way of being. The secret is to be consistent for the ten-day period, allow this time to begin to dissolve old patterns, which in turn will give you a whole new perspective on dealing with stress. Equally, if you decide to give up chocolate or coffee for the ten-day period, you will have a much clearer understanding of the effect when, in the future, you have a cup of coffee or a bar of chocolate.

Conclusion

I believe that a programme of change is like a journey in three stages. I like to use the analogy of blasting off from Cape Canaveral to the moon. Basically this journey has three important stages.

1　Blast off. This is where you initiate the programme. You sit very tight in your seat in the capsule, you have read the manual carefully, you are following the advice from Mission Control and, as you gain momentum and hurtle towards space, there is little opportunity to wave, meander or even think very much. The main thing is that you trust what you are doing and that you remain focused on your destination – the moon.

2　This is the unpleasant stage when you pass through the earth's atmosphere. You still remain firmly in your seat and try not to be distracted by the new sensations, new noises and unpleasant turbulence. This parallels the experience of elimination that I mentioned previously.

3　Once you exit the earth's orbit and are clearly on target for the moon you can get out of your seat, relax, eat, take in the view, do your work and, because the pressure and speed of change has slowed down considerably, you can afford to meander a little off target. In fact, no space craft flies in a straight line. It veers to the left or right and, with a little boost here and there from the rockets, you can be back on course again.

In summing up the best advice is to remain centred, focused and on target for the initial few days, ride through the ups and downs and then relax and begin to use your own pilotage skills – enjoy.

Step One: Knowing Who and Where You Are

The self-assessment questions that now follow give you the opportunity to use the unique and time-tested system of oriental diagnosis to assess your current situation. In the first instance, you will be able to determine whether your overall constitution – your capacity and innate potential – is primarily yin or yang. Remember that our constitution never changes and by determining this factor it is possible to get a bearing on how you are likely to go about your work and recreation.

The second part of the questionnaire deals primarily with your current condition. You will be able to use this section time and time again as our condition is in a constant state of flux. Run through the checklist in the different sections, ticking off where you feel you identify most with the statements and then see which way your current condition is leaning and to what degree. Finally, prioritize the areas in your life where you feel a desire for change. By the end of this chapter you will be clear about knowing your constitution (who you are), your current condition (where you are) and the priorities that you have selected in areas of your life that you wish to focus on in the ten-day programme.

WHO YOU ARE (constitution)

Running through the checklist below, tick off the boxes that you feel are appropriate. At the end of this section note whether there is a swing toward yin or yang.

Bone structure

Would you consider yourself to have a heavy or light bone structure? You can often notice this in the bones of the wrist and the ankle. Do they appear delicate or robust compared with other men or women of your age and ethnic group? Remember that underlying bone structure is constitutional whereas body weight is conditional.

	Yin	Yang
Heavy		☑
Light	☐	

Relative to your family and other members of your ethnic group, would you consider yourself tall or short?

	Yin	Yang
Tall	☑	
Short		☐

Face shape

You may find yourself having to look at other faces around you before you can determine the distinction between square, round, long and thin! Perhaps glance through a current magazine and look at twenty to thirty different faces, then it is not difficult to notice the distinction. A square head can incorporate a broad brow and a square jaw, whereas a round face can include a softer jaw and a little more of a dome to the top of the head. A long face can have a high forehead and a longer chin. A thin face shape can also be described as a narrow face where the eyes are fairly close together, the nose is narrow and the chin and jaw area also narrow.

	Yin	Yang
Square		☐
Round		☑
Long	☐	
Thin	☐	

Jaw

Look at your jaw and chin and note whether it is square, thick-set or more narrow leading towards a point:

	Yin	Yang
Square jaw		☐
Pointed jaw	☐	

Head:body ratio

You will need to look at yourself in a photograph or a full-length mirror to determine the size of your head relative to the rest of your body. Again, you may need to look at several photographs in a magazine or observe others for a short while to get a comparison.

	Yin	Yang
Head relatively large compared to the size of your body		☐
Head relatively small compared to the size of your body	☐	

Hands

Have a close look at the palms of your hands and determine whether the shape is more square or elongated. An easy way to do this is to examine the palm of your left hand and use your thumb and middle finger from your right hand as a pair of dividers. Measure across the palm in one direction (from the edge to the base of the thumb). Now use those same 'dividers' to measure from the base of the wrist to the beginning of the fingers. If the distance is the same you have square palms, if the palm is narrow you have long palms.

	Yin	Yang
Square		☐
Long	☐	

Are your fingers long or short? Measure the distance between the base of your wrist and where your fingers begin. Using this same measurement notice whether your middle finger is approximately the same length. If your fingers are considerably shorter than this distance and are relatively thick and stubby then you have short fingers. If your fingers are thin and with the fingers of your hand closed and held up to the light you can see gaps between them then consider your fingers as long.

	Yin	Yang
Long	☐	
Short		☐

Ears

Again, you may need to look at other members of your family or colleagues to determine the relative sizes and differences that appear in ear shapes. The shape and size of our ears can provide us one of the most accurate insights into the nature of our constitution.

	Yin	Yang
Big		☐
Small	☐	
Fleshy		☐
Lean	☐	

Teeth

The overall health and strength of our teeth is – like that of our bones – a very good indication of inherent constitution. The simplest way of assessing them is to determine whether they are strong or weak. Strong means that you are capable of cracking nuts and have very few dental problems. Weak teeth chip easily and over the years you have needed plenty of specialist dental care.

	Yin	Yang
Strong		☐
Weak	☐	

Conclusion

Count up the number of yins and yangs in the preceding questionnaire.

Do you consider your constitution to be more:

Yin ☐

or more

Yang ☐

Yin constitution

If you have identified yourself as having an intrinsic yin nature then these are some of the traits that can be associated: intellectual, perceptive, thoughtful, watchful, cautious, calm, artistic, elegant, critical, delicate, sensitive, dreamer, compassionate, nimble, sprightly.

Yang constitution

If you have identified yourself as having a more yang nature, here are some of the traits that have a leaning toward yang: adventurous, frank, practical, pragmatic, astute, impulsive, bold, boisterous, jovial, robust, rebellious, enthusiastic, methodical.

WHERE YOU ARE (condition)

Since our condition is constantly changing you can fall back on the following questionnaire time and time again. The method of oriental diagnosis used here is the most practical for you to use on yourself. If you feel that you do not identify with any of the traits listed below, simply do not tick any box, but if several are apt you may tick more than one in any section. At the end of the questionnaire just add up how many 'yins' and 'yangs' you have collected and note your score.

How do you feel?

Please tick one or more of the following four categories if they are realistically fairly dominant in how you feel at the current time. Tiredness implies that fatigue is present throughout much of the day. Hyperactivity means that you find it normal to be on the go all the time. Difficulty relaxing can be expressed as the inability to 'switch off' or to be drawn to any form of recreation. Difficulty getting motivated relates to an indifference to social entertainment as well to completing a project or starting something fresh.

	Yin	Yang
Tiredness	☐	
Hyperactivity		☐
Difficulty relaxing		☐
Difficulty getting motivated	☐	

Behaviour

Do you currently find yourself taking a very rigid or inflexible stance about your own opinions or inflexible to change? Do you think that others are finding you unreasonably demanding or pushy at the current time? Are you on the other hand becoming more forgetful or constantly changing your mind?

	Yin	Yang
Inflexible to change		☐
Increasingly demanding		☐

Do you find others unreasonably
demanding or pushy ☐

Forgetful or constantly
changing your mind ☐

Sleep

Your sleep pattern is an excellent indication of whether your current condition is more yin or more yang. The more sleep you need the more yin you are, the less the more yang at present. Excessively yin would be nine hours plus and excessively yang is less than six.

	Yin	Yang
More than 9 hours	☐	
Less than 6 hours		☐

Urination

Traditional Chinese medicine and pre-20th century Western medicine both held the view that the quality and output of urine was always an indication of an individual's current condition. Go through the following checklist and see if any of these symptoms are noticeable and remember that they can change on an almost daily basis. On frequency it is important to take into account whether you have an unusually small bladder. The normal frequency of passing urine is four to five times daily, colour like a light beer and a mild odour.

	Yin	Yang
Do you urinate often?	☐	
Infrequently?		☐
Is your urine dark?		☐
Is your urine clear?	☐	
Strong odour		☐
Little or no odour	☐	

Bowels

Stools are always examined for their size, odour and frequency in the Far East, as they were in pre-20th century Western medicine. Normal could be considered as: at least one bowel movement a day, mild odour, gold in colour. A good indication of whether the stools are hard or loose is the amount of toilet tissue you require. Half a roll is too loose, none at all too hard.

	Yin	Yang
Bowels loose	☐	
Bowels hard		☐
Light colour	☐	
Dark colour		☐
Bowel movements frequent (2-3 x day)	☐	
Bowel movements infrequent (2-3 x week)		☐

Voice

The quality, depth and rhythm of your voice is an accurate barometer of your current condition. See where you sit within these six different categories.

	Yin	Yang
Loud		☐
Soft	☐	
High	☐	
Low		☐
Clear		☐
Weak	☐	

Handwriting

Simply put pen to paper and write a couple of sentences and see how your writing appears today. Spidery writing implies that your hand may be trembling slightly or weak. A lack of pressure (soft) or an incompleteness (where the strokes seem to tail off) are all yin indications. However, deep pressure on the pad or fast, bold strokes of the pen indicate that your current condition is more yang.

	Yin	Yang
Spidery	☐	
Soft/incomplete	☐	
Bold		☐
Deep pressure		☐

Walking

Be aware of how you move around today. Do you move very quickly and directly? Are you walking slowly, often distracted by a shop window or otherwise easily diverted? When in a crowded area are you patient or impatient and determined?

	Yin	Yang
Purposeful/fast		☐
Slow/meandering	☐	
Patient	☐	
Impatient		☐

Muscles

Your muscle tone doesn't change overnight but it does relate well to whether your overall current condition is leaning towards yin or yang. Do take into account whether you have taken any strong, strenuous exercise in the past forty-eight hours. This may well have left you with some pain in your muscles.

	Yin	Yang
Is your grip weak?	☐	
Is your grip vice-like?		☐
Do you have any dull aches in muscles?	☐	
Do you have any sharp pain in muscles?		☐

Do you feel very tense?	☐
Do you feel too loose?	☐

Skin

Your skin, rather like your digestive and elimination systems, is a good indicator of your overall health. The dryer and more leathery the skin the more yang we are, the more oily or 'puffy' the more yin.

	Yin	Yang
Does your skin look old/ withered (considering your age)		☐
Is your skin puffy?	☐	
Is your skin oily?	☐	
Is your skin dry?		☐

Eyes

Undoubtedly the most profound indication as to whether your condition is excessively yin or yang would be the discovery that you were san paku (see pp. 79-80). In my opinion this one method of diagnosis is enough to assess whether our condition is extremely yin or extremely yang. However, it is quite likely that you will be neither yin nor yang san paku as this reflects a large swing towards an extreme condition.

Do your eyes appear tired or bright? Do you notice that you are staring intensely at the moment or do your eyes tend to wander and drift? We normally blink approximately three times every minute, a lot more than this and your condition is more yin, a lot less (once or perhaps twice a minute) and your condition is definitely yang.

	Yin	Yang
Yin san paku	☐	
Yang san paku		☐
Eyes tired	☐	
Eyes bright		☐
Blink frequently	☐	
Blink infrequently		☐
A tendency to stare		☐
A tendency to drift	☐	

Hair

You may have noticed in the past, when you felt run down or had a cold, your hair becomes more yin – limp, damp or oily. See how your hair feels at the moment. You can judge this by the frequency that you need to wash your hair, its manageability and how it appears first thing in the morning.

	Yin	Yang
Hair damp/oily	☐	
Hair dry		☐
Hair limp	☐	
Hair undisciplined		☐

Tongue

You need only to glimpse your tongue to make this assessment. Make sure there is good lighting near the mirror and avoid making your tongue tense. Simply let it hang loose and for no more than ten seconds at a time. Remember that a normal tongue will be moist, the colour of fresh meat and with a very pale coating.

	Yin	Yang
Is your tongue wet?	☐	
Is your tongue dry?		☐
Is your tongue pale/white?	☐	
Is your tongue red/yellow?		☐

Pulse

Check back to p. 82 for guidance in taking your pulse and use any of the three middle fingers to locate it. Remember that a normal pulse is four beats per respiration. Slower than this and you are more yin, faster than this and you are yang. Obviously the most practical time of day to take this reading is when you get up or are reasonably sedentary.

	Yin	Yang
Pulse slow (up to 4 beats/resp)	☐	
Pulse fast (more than 4 beats/resp)		☐
Pulse soft	☐	
Pulse throbbing		☐

Conclusion

Count up your answers. How do you rate your overall condition today?

Yin ☐

Yang ☐

Now please read through the following six sections and see if you identify with any of the areas. Look for signs or symptoms where you feel you could be operating better. Tick as many areas as you wish.

Activity

This relates to your day-to-day activity – whether it is your work or your creativity. How do you rate yourself in relationships with others at present? What feedback have you had from your partner in terms of your sex life? What kind of recreational activities are you drawn to at present? How do you go about them?

	Yin	Yang
Slow	☐	
Fast		☐
Quiet	☐	
Loud		☐
Passive	☐	
Aggressive		☐

Lacking in self esteem ☐

Over confident ☐

Indifferent ☐

Competitive ☐

Concerning activity are you:

Yin ☐

or

Yang ☐

Stress

Look at the list below and see if you can identify any of the physical or emotional traits that are either more yin or more yang. Simply add up your score and notice whether your stress is related to your condition being more yin or more yang.

Yin symptoms of stress

Constantly late for meetings or friends ☐

Tendency to procrastinate ☐

Feeling that you are losing control ☐

Finding yourself in tears frequently ☐

Feeling in a panic ☐

Starting to withdraw from friends
or colleagues ☐

A general feeling of helplessness ☐

A tendency while under stress toward
rapid breathing ☐

General fatigue ☐

A trembling sensation in your hands,
face or feet ☐

Being more susceptible to colds/flu
or infections ☐

The desire to urinate more frequently ☐

Yang symptoms of stress

Inability to sleep (insomnia) ☐

Pain in the side or back of the neck ☐

Increased irritability ☐

Unusual displays of aggressiveness ☐

Feeling constantly restless ☐

A tendency to frown ☐

Clenching your teeth ☐

Unusually excited over small occurrences ☐

Increasingly impulsive ☐

Impatient with those around you ☐

Do you pace up and down like a
caged animal? ☐

Under pressure do you tap your fingers on
the table or keep moving your foot or leg?   ☐

How do you rate your stress levels?
Are you dominantly:

Yin   ☐

or

Yang   ☐

Environment

For this part of the programme you need to concentrate on
where your own energy and health is recharged and revitalized
on a daily basis – your home. Next time you enter your space
after a day out or at work, use this list to help you notice it from
a more objective angle. How does it 'feel' to you? Is it warm and
inviting? Is it cold? If at the end of this section you feel that the
space has too much of a yang or yin effect, there will be recommendations for you in Chapter 8.

Too much yin in your environment:

Large space   ☐

Dark   ☐

Cold   ☐

Old   ☐

Damp   ☐

Lack of air or plant life   ☐

Do you use a lot of electrical gadgetry in your cooking e.g. microwaves, electric cooker, freezer? ☐

Do you feel isolated? ☐

Do you feel unmotivated when in the space? ☐

Too much yang in your environment:

Is it a small space (cramped)? ☐

Is the lighting too bright and glaring? ☐

Is it very hot? ☐

Is it very modern? ☐

Does it feel dry or arid? ☐

Is there a lack of softness in the furnishings and colours? ☐

Do you have a lot of modern technology e.g. computers, etc. ☐

Do you feel busy in this space? ☐

Do you find it difficult to relax in this space? ☐

Overall, is the impression that your space has a strong:

Yin effect ☐

or a

Yang effect ☐

Patterns of behaviour

Look at the following columns and honestly declare whether any of these patterns of behaviour are starting to emerge. If you find that four or five of them appear in one of the sections then it is well worth looking at ways to redress the balance during this ten-day period outlined in Chapter 8.

Yin patterns of behaviour:

Are you finding yourself complaining more than usual? ☐

Are you beginning to display a loss of ambition? ☐

Are you beginning to lose your self-confidence? ☐

Are you becoming increasingly forgetful? ☐

Are you becoming unnecessarily fearful? ☐

Are you becoming more defensive? ☐

Are you becoming more suspicious or sceptical? ☐

Are you finding yourself retreating into yourself or your space? ☐

Are you displaying signs of an inferiority complex? ☐

Are you beginning to live in a world of fantasy or illusion? ☐

Do you feel yourself a victim? ☐

Yang patterns of behaviour:

Are you becoming rigid in your outlook
and your approach to life? ☐

Are you becoming stubborn? ☐

Do you find yourself becoming caught up
in trivial matters and detail? ☐

Are you becoming unusually excitable? ☐

Do you find yourself becoming more
offensive? ☐

Do you have less tolerance to others and
are more prone to lose your temper? ☐

Are you showing signs of prejudice and
discrimination? ☐

Are you becoming exclusive – in your beliefs
or in who you wish to be associated with? ☐

Do you have a superiority complex? ☐

Are you becoming self-righteous? ☐

Are you becoming more forceful and
controlling? ☐

Are you becoming increasingly egocentric
or selfish? ☐

Do the patterns of behaviour show that you are:

More yin ☐

or

More yang ☐

Spirit/Chi

Our Chi simply reflects how we are feeling at the moment. This is an important area to analyse and very easy to turn around with the ideas outlined in Chapter 8.

Yin qualities of our Chi include:

Being cautious ☐

Going with the flow/crowd ☐

Staying up late ☐

Difficulty waking up ☐

Feeling isolated or out of touch ☐

Yang qualities of our Chi include:

Being criticized for insensitivity ☐

Being currently hyperactive/workaholic ☐

Difficulty relaxing ☐

Increasingly impatient ☐

Little need for sleep or rest ☐

How do you rate your Chi at present:

More yin   ☐

or

More yang   ☐

Diet

Take a moment to go through the list of ingredients below.
They include the more extreme ends of the food spectrums.
Simply tick a box if you use any of these products more than
three or four times a week. If you never use any of these products
you can skip this exercise, but it is perhaps still worth doing if
you only indulge in any of them even once or twice a week.

Strong yin factors within the diet include:

White sugar		☐
Sorbitol	}	
Saccharin	}	
Nutra-sweet	}	☐
Brown sugar	}	
Glucose	}	
Honey		☐
Chocolate		☐
Ice-cream		☐
Milk		☐

Yoghurt ☐

Cream and soft dairy products ☐

Coffee ☐

Aromatic and commercial teas ☐

Cola ☐

Pepper ☐

Tropical fruits ☐

Raw tropical nuts ☐

Tomatoes ☐

Potatoes ☐

White flour products ☐

Fruit based alcohol (wine, sherry, port, brandy, champagne and cider) ☐

Yang dietary factors include:

Eggs (include hidden eggs in baking, etc.) ☐

Fish roe (including caviar) ☐

Beef ☐

Lamb ☐

Pork ☐

Ham ☐

Sausage ☐

Bacon ☐

Game ☐

Pâté ☐

Chicken ☐

Duck ☐

Turkey ☐

Salmon ☐

Tuna ☐

Refined salt ☐

Cheese (hard or cooked) ☐

Soya sauce ☐

Did you find that your diet was predominant in:

Yin factors ☐

or

Yang factors ☐

Conclusion

Congratulations for working your way through this self-assessment checklist. I hope that it has not left you neurotic but potentially inspired to bring about some kind of change. At this stage of the game it is worth prioritizing one or two areas of your life that you wish to focus on. Choose those you have ticked the most in the sub-sections.

Below are the six areas where you could begin to work. Tick the appropriate box(es) and keep the areas you choose on hold at the back of your mind as you move to the next stage of the programme. There is no need to tick a box in every line.

	Too Yin	Too Yang
Activity	☐	☐
Stress	☐	☐
Environment	☐	☐
Patterns and behaviour	☐	☐
Spirit/Chi	☐	☐
Diet	☐	☐

7

Step Two: Planning the Voyage

THE POWER OF THE MIND

For the next step in bringing about any change in your life, you need to have a clear idea as to what you want to achieve. The mind, and the clarity of our intuition, play important roles in making that goal both practical and clear. During this unique ten-day period you will have the opportunity to steer a clear path through the normal day-to-day distractions and begin to focus on your dream. Our mind has the potential to give us the will and inspiration to make and see through changes, but equally it can provide us with all the stumbling blocks for effectively maintaining a status quo.

We are all aware of the positive effect that, for example, encouragement can have, whether it is from a colleague or a coach. The feeling of being acknowledged or supported has a very powerful effect on our frame of mind. On the other hand, criticism from others and our own negative self-talk can completely block our route to change. Much of this negative self-talk is ingrained in us at an early, impressionable age. Frequently, many of our failures in adult life can be attributed to a lingering yet unconscious memory of criticism or prediction of failure received in childhood. These unconscious 'blocks' that are imprinted in our minds can include: 'I am a failure,' I am useless,' 'I am not intelligent enough,' 'I am not athletic enough,' 'I am a slob,' 'I am a waste of time,' 'I am a waste of space' – and so the list goes on. Most analysts would agree that three major factors that occur in our childhood during a particular event help to fashion and harden these inner statements.

1 At the time you must have been in a state of great vulnerability. You were under abnormal pressure, you were very worried and possibly fearful. The classic scenario would have been having your back against the wall in a situation where there was no escape and no opportunity to defend yourself or to reason with the person sharing the confrontation.

2 At the same time the person that you were in conflict with had a particularly domineering nature. They were overbearing, they were bigger than you, older and certainly in authority over you at the time. This person could have been a bully, an irate parent, a very angry or domineering teacher, an insensitive doctor, or some officer of the law.

3 The final ingredient within this scenario, to complete the imprinting, would be this person forecasting some kind of future for you. It was probably not meant maliciously but it left you with a sense of foreboding that is deeply ingrained. Many kinds of therapy attempt to work back in time to discover the nature of this forecast and to help you invent a new life based on a new-found sense of freedom and self-expression. Left unattended, however, one wonders how many people are unconsciously living out a prophecy that was made when they were young.

Some of the common forecasts that are revealed include: 'You will never be big and strong like your brother,' 'If you don't eat your food you will fade away,' 'Your life will not be worth living,' 'You will always be in trouble,' 'You will be the cause of my undoing.' In the section headed 'Patterns of Behaviour' of Chapter 8 there are some useful exercises which are designed to help you to reflect upon and release these ingrained patterns.

To get the most from this section on visualization, remind

yourself of the enormous creative potential of the mind. To put this potential in perspective, try to remember that there are three areas that you could explore:

- What you are capable of. Defining this area means knowing what we know and equally knowing our limitations in terms of skill, knowledge and practice.
- What you *could* be capable of. All of us are aware that there are areas of knowledge that, should we choose to find out, we could grasp. For example, we are aware that there is an enormous body of knowledge about flying and navigation. We do not necessarily know anything about the subject but, should we choose to, it would be relatively simple to find out more.
- What you are not even aware you could be capable of. The first two areas are relatively simple to understand – what you know and what you know you could find out about. However, this third area is exciting new territory: areas of knowledge, practice, study or potential of which we are not even aware let alone have begun to tap into. This is the realm of dreams! It is in this area that the ensuing section on visualization helps you. Imagine predicting in 1980 that within a few years communism would collapse in Russia and much of the Eastern Bloc? Imagine predicting at the same time that within a few years the communist party would be legal in South Africa. Nelson Mandela would be free and the republic's president. Imagine also in 1980 predicting that the Berlin Wall would come down – not by an act of war but by the overwhelming power of people's will and desire for change? It is accessing the special dream that each of us has, unhindered by any negative self-talk or critique by others, that is the essence of this powerful visualization exercise.

Martin Luther King's speech of 28 August 1963 to 210,000

people in Washington drew on much the same flavour when he declared:

> I have a dream that one day this nation will rise up and live out the true meaning of its creed: we hold these truths to be self-evident: that all men are created equal.
>
> I have a dream that one day on the red hills of Georgia the sons of former slaves and the sons of former state owners will be able to sit down together at the table of brotherhood.
>
> I have a dream that one day even the state of Mississippi, the desert state sweltering with the heat of injustice and oppression, will be transformed into an oasis of freedom and justice.
>
> I have a dream that my four little children will one day live in a nation where they will not be judged by the colour of their skin but by the content of their character.
>
> I have a dream today.

Visualization

In terms of yin and yang, the world of dreams, planning and the future is yin. Left unattended this would remain out there in the atmosphere – a vibration, a thought, something intangible. However, harness that dream, give it some focus, give it some legs, give it some muscle and give it a direction (all of them yang factors) and you have a potentially far more creative proposition. If you have never done any visualization work or are very sceptical about it or feel that there is little connection between our mind and our body, then I would like you to try this simple exercise.

You need to sit quietly for a moment with your eyes closed, allow your breathing to become still and to centre it in your abdomen. Don't worry about the distractions of your mind, just maintain a simple stillness. Now imagine this. See yourself pick up a very fresh lime or lemon from a plate on a table in front of you. See yourself peel the skin of this fruit with your fingernails or a knife. Then see yourself pick up this fruit and bite deeply into it so that at least half of the fruit is in your mouth. See yourself chew the fruit and get in touch at this stage with the sensations it is producing physically within your mouth. Give it a go!

On some level I am sure you had a response! You may have felt great trepidation about putting raw lime or lemon into your mouth and chewing it. Equally, in anticipation your mouth may have begun to water. If you have very good imagination then as you began to bite into and consequently chew this acidic fruit it would have left your mouth and even your eyes watering. It is a simple but very effective exercise showing the connection between your mind and your body.

To get the most out of visualization we need to shift from a mode of 'doing' to a mode of 'being'. Essentially this means that we need time to be still, quiet, relaxed and completely undistracted. There is little point in practising the exercise I am about to describe while travelling on public transport. This isn't an attempt, like some form of meditation, to help you achieve a state of relaxed well-being. It is much more about seeing yourself and how you are being in the future. The practical use of visualization in Western culture is very grounded and pragmatic. I think a very good example of it is the so-called business plan. Ask a friend or colleague involved in economics whether their company has a business plan. Inevitably the company does and from my research these plans can be fairly detailed, up to five years ahead and, to some extent, with less detail, up to fifteen years. It's a very different situation in the Far East – especially in Japan. Privately, I have been told that many Japanese banks and stockbroking firms have business plans – they are indeed as detailed as those of any Western financial institutions in terms of the next five to fifteen years. However, the difference is that they also have a 'dream'. This dream may only reside with top members of the board and it may not necessarily go into great detail about the financial figures, but it certainly has a lot to do with forward planning and policy, into a future that will far outlive the current directors. The benefit of having a long-term game plan or dream is that you can build in allowances for hiccup, failure or losses as well as surges for growth at the same time. It is holding this long-term 'dream' in place that is the purpose of the visualization exercise that I invite you to try.

The visualization exercise

This exercise can bring you to a unique point where you will be capable of imagining yourself and even possibly seeing yourself at some point in the future. It is up to you to decide whether that future is a week ahead, a month, a year, five years or even longer.

The difference between this exercise and others is the potential to begin to 'live into' the dream that it produces almost immediately. If you see yourself in the future as someone who is successful in a particular field, start to believe and be that now. When you begin to change your vibration – your Chi - that bright, new, optimistic 'successful' Chi will begin to emanate from you. That in turn will have two powerful effects. Firstly, it will begin to pull you towards realizing your dream and secondly, others will notice your new-found Chi. It then has the potential to manifest not only in your behaviour and body language but also in how you go about your daily life. Instead of thinking: 'I will be successful in three years' time,' it translates into 'I am successful now.' You may not achieve the level of success that you wish overnight, but you and your dream are now united by an imaginary piece of elastic that is drawing you ever closer towards that reality.

My advice for the first attempt at this particular exercise is to see what unfolds in the visualization and then to undertake practical steps that will have measurable results for you within the next ten days. Remember that you can fall back on this exercise at any time, and that if this is your first attempt at visualization you don't *have* to 'do' anything. It is far more a question of being in the moment and allowing whatever unfolds to unfold.

Naturally, keep in the back of your mind at the start of the exercise the priorities in your life where you are looking to make changes. This gives the process a little more focus and direction. If you have a more yin nature you will find it easy to 'dream' and may need to be clearer at the beginning of the exercise which area(s) of your life you are visualizing. Conversely, more 'yang' individuals are more pragmatic and may 'try' too hard to make something happen. It is best for them to relax and allow the process to be more spontaneous.

How to do the visualization

The actual length of time that your eyes are closed and that you are 'being' with the exercise can be as little as three to ten minutes. But to benefit most from the exercise I encourage you to put aside a period of at least twenty to thirty minutes when you know you will not be disturbed. This allows you plenty of time to relax, settle into the visualization and be with the visualization for three to ten minutes, a few minutes to relax and come out of the visualization and then a few more minutes to go through the questionnaire and complete the various steps outlined.

Set out below are the guidelines for the step-by-step approach. You could either a) read through the guidelines several times so that you are familiar with the various steps and stages and then, when you are ready, put them into practice. Or b) ask a close friend who is sensitive to what you are trying to achieve to read through the guidelines while you are practising the visualization. They need to read through the guidelines a couple of times first, to familiarize themselves with the routine. This second method can be very effective as you are completely unencumbered by time or trying to remember what to do next.

In any event when you feel the 'dream' or the image starting to fade or becoming too mechanical it is time to wind down and return to the room.

Guidelines

1 Be sure that you can be uninterrupted for about thirty
   minutes. Put the telephone on ansaphone, perhaps have
   some quiet background music playing, without lyrics. I
   prefer to do this exercise while sitting comfortably rather
   than lying down as your Chi is likely to be more focused
   when you are upright.

2 Close your eyes and be aware of your breathing. Bring
   your breathing down into your belly until you are aware
   that your abdomen is gently expanding and contracting as
   you breathe.

3 To deeply and fully relax your body the following
   exercise is very helpful. On each out breath imagine that
   you are turning off a light switch which is associated with
   a different part of your body. Beginning with the head,
   neck and shoulders and working all the way down towards
   the toes, this exercise can leave you deeply relaxed. As you
   breathe out imagine switching off the switch connected to
   the muscles around your eyes, on the next breath out
   switch off the jaw, on the next the neck, on the next
   switch off the shoulders, on the next the right arm, elbow,
   wrist and hand. Then, on the next out breath switch off
   the left arm, elbow, wrist and hand. As you breathe out
   switch off the chest, on the next breath switch off the
   abdomen, and on the next switch off the pelvis, on the
   next the right leg, knee, calf and foot, and on the last out
   breath switch off the left leg, knee, calf and foot. You will
   now be physically relaxed. Now allow yourself to 'be'.
   Sometimes it is beneficial to imagine yourself in a special
   place that has inspired you and that has a natural
   environment. It could be where you recently spent a
   holiday or watched a sunset or somewhere you recall
   from your childhood. Try not to make anything happen.

4 If you feel any negative emotions arise or tensions or
   strange sensations in your body that begin to distract you,

allow them to bubble up and out through your exhalation to let them dissipate. Try not to linger on them, encounter them or diagnose them in any way. Just be with the feelings and sensations and allow the out breath to dissolve them.

5 Soon you will find yourself in a very relaxed space and can allow yourself to dream and imagine yourself at some point in the future. As images come and go try to recall some of them for the later part of the exercise. But try not to make anything specific happen; enjoy the power and potential of your imagination and ultimately enjoy it. Wallow in your fantasy!

6 Hopefully, you will have caught a glimpse of yourself – where you are or what you are doing, how you are being in the future. When the images begin to get fuzzy or you notice yourself becoming more mechanical and conscious, it is time to return to the present.

7 Continue sitting comfortably, allowing your breath to be deep and from the abdomen and 'switch on' your body in reverse order. As you breathe in, turn on the switches in your left leg, calf, knee and foot. Then as you breathe in, the switch in your right leg, calf, knee and foot. Turn on the switch in your pelvis, then your abdomen and then your chest. Turn on the switches in your left hand, elbow and arm. As you breathe in, turn on your right hand, elbow and arm, then your shoulder, neck and jaw, and finally turn on the switches behind and around the eyes.

8 Begin to wriggle your fingers and your toes and slowly open your eyes.

9 As soon as you are alert enough take up your pad and pencil and scribble down as much detail as possible of what you saw. Note any emotions or sensations that you felt. What did you sense you were doing in the future? How did you feel about what you were doing and how you were being? Try to get down as soon as possible as much information as you can recall.

The conscious reality – living into the dream

a) The dream

The next stage of this exercise is to take yourself from the 'big picture' of what you saw possible down through the detail of what you can begin to put into place today. Take a moment to reflect on how you saw yourself, what you were doing, your surroundings, who you were with, how you were being and how you felt. When you have a sense of the future in which you saw yourself you can begin to make note of some of the details that you observed. When I first did this exercise some ten years ago I was living in a confined urban environment with a young family. I saw myself and my family living in the country, with plenty of space, near the sea and in a house that was detached from its neighbours with plenty of space for the children to play. I also saw myself working part-time from home with occasional commutes into London. At the time of the exercise, I took notes and later even gave them more boldness by typing them and adding a statement of my dream. Within a year we had moved to the country and almost all of the dream had fallen into place. It was only the areas that I was unclear about or had not been specific about that came to be a cause of distraction in the future.

While you are still enjoying a more reflective state, please begin to work on the following declaration:
'Who I am is . . .'

It is best to avoid a statement such as 'Who I will be . . .' It is far more powerful to declare now who you are. You can begin to 'be' that vision rather than dreaming that it is somewhere down the line.

A very short while ago, I did this exercise with a group of students in Belgium. At that point in my life I was unclear whether I would continue as a lecturer and a counsellor or perhaps try my hand at a different approach to self-healing. I had given some thought to the possibility of writing. My logical mind gave me all the indications that it was not possible. I had no experience. I did not have a publisher. It was new territory. Would anybody be interested? The list was endless. However, while leading the students through the visualization exercise I was participating myself. I was completely open to seeing and being what I saw myself as in the future. I saw myself on a stage in a very smart cream suit completing a presentation on self-healing. I saw several piles of books in front of me in a warm, comfortable room and I felt confident and encouraged by the audience. At the end of the visualization, the students gave their feedback as to who they saw themselves, and they were genuinely committed to making that possible as each declared who they were. I declared myself not just an author but a SUCCESSFUL author. After the lecture I told my wife that who I was, was a successful author, and she turned to me in a very matter-of-fact down-to-earth Croation manner and said 'of course you are, dear!'

b) The commitment

Now we need to examine what can fire you up to realize your dream at the present moment. What do you need to change in terms of your attitude and outlook to make it possible? There needs to be some shift in how you go about your day-to-day business in order to make this dream possible. What is your new stand? What is your new position? How would you communicate this to others both verbally and in your actions? Keep this perspective fairly broad at present, but you do need to declare some statement of new policy that you can begin to be and live into.

Examples of how you could phrase this include:

'I am committed to losing weight'
'I am committed to gaining weight'
'I am committed to having an attractive body'
'I am committed to being more flexible'
'I am committed to having more stamina'

'I am committed to owning a beautiful new home'
'I am committed to regular holidays'
'I am committed to a wonderful relationship'
'I am committed to take more time for myself'
'I am committed to give more support to my family'
'I am committed to having more fun'
'I am committed to taking life more seriously'

Here is your opportunity to declare your new policy – keeping it broad, as the opportunity to fill in the detail will appear later in this exercise.

'I am committed to . . .'

c) The intention

Now that you have declared your dream and begun to shape your policy it is time to be clear about which area(s) of your life you intend to bring changes into. The information in Chapter 8 will give you plenty of practical insights, ideas and support for changes in the following categories:

1 Activity – looking at your work, your recreation and how you go about your daily business.
2 Stress – how you are coping with the pressures of your lifestyle, your work and your relationships.
3 Environment – making practical changes in your home to bring freshness, vitality and even relaxation.
4 Patterns of behaviour – an opportunity to bring about and initiate changes in 'how you are being', to help you reflect on whether you are repeating the same patterns over and over again.
5 Spirit/Chi – are there areas in your overall energy that have become hyperactive or stagnant and where you could benefit from changing or harnessing in a creative way?
6 Diet – are there changes that you could make in what you

eat, how it is prepared, the attention you pay to chewing and appreciating your food?

Remember that all of these areas are in essence connected. However, take on one or two, perhaps three of the categories and begin to declare your intention of the area that you wish to work on. For example, you could declare:

'I intend to take on more physical activity'
or –
'I intend to get involved socially with sport'
or –
'I intend to learn to meditate'
or –
'I intend to take up yoga'
or –
'I intend to bring about changes in my home'
or –
'I intend to change my diet'
or –
'I intend to socialize more'
or –
'I intend to complete all that I undertake'
etc, etc, etc.

At this stage in the process you need to complete this declaration:
'I intend to . . .'

d) The game plan

Now that you have a sense of the areas of your life that you wish to work on, begin to be a little more specific about what you wish to undertake in that particular category. Below are six areas that we will concentrate on in Chapter 8. Read through the points and, if you wish, fill in the space for each section at its head. You may list more than one or you may skip a section.

- Activity

I need . . .

> to slow down
> or –
> to become more relaxed
> or –
> more physical activity
> or –
> more fresh air
> or –
> to play more sports with other people

- Stress

I need . . .

> to learn visualization exercises to help me relax
> or –
> to have a regular massage
> or –
> to learn aromatherapy
> or –
> to learn Tai Chi
> or –
> to learn how to release my tension
> or –
> to learn how to focus my energy

- Environment

I need to bring . . .

> more brightness into my home
> or –
> more colour into my home

or –
more air into my home
or –
more life into my home
or –
more warmth into my home
or –
more relaxation into my home

- Patterns of behaviour

I need . . .

to take more risks
or –
to socialize more
or –
to develop my self-expression
or –
to stand up for myself
or –
to listen more to others
or –
to show my feelings
or –
to release my anger
or –
to release my resentment

- Spirit/Chi

I need . . .

to get up earlier
or –
to slow down
or –
to take a holiday

or –
more sleep
or –
to develop my softer side
or –
to develop more aggression
or –
to become more competitive

- Diet

I need . . .

more freshness in my food
or –
to be more aware of what I am eating
or –
to eat good quality food
or –
to cook my own food
or –
more variety in my cooking styles
or –
more 'fire' in my food
or –
more 'relaxing' foods

Priorities

Have a look at the points you have picked above and see if there are areas you feel you should focus on. You can complete this stage of the exercise by declaring that you need to take action in the following areas: Activity, Stress, Environment, Patterns of Behaviour, Spirit/Chi and Diet, and ideally choose only one or two, certainly no more than four.

-
-
-
-

e) The first steps

Bearing in mind how you see yourself in the future and what you wish to achieve, begin to be very specific as to what you will guarantee to initiate or undertake as of NOW. Create a 'to do' list. What are the tasks you need to undertake today to get the ball rolling? It is pointless having a grand vision without setting into place the mechanical steps for bringing it about. Remember to be very specific and precise – these can be small steps at this stage. Keep it simple and at the same time make it achievable and practical.

For example, you could declare that today you will begin to chew your food more slowly and thoroughly. Perhaps you will clean and tidy your kitchen this evening. It could be that you decide to buy a book on Tai Chi or investigate where you can learn meditation at a local evening class. You could telephone a friend and agree to go out to the cinema next week or book a game of squash with a colleague. Whatever it is, don't put it off until tomorrow but make a list of what you will undertake TODAY:

-
-
-
-
-
-

-
-
-
-

There are plenty of ideas and suggestions coming up in the next chapter that you may choose to add. They are primarily designed to initiate a shift from symptoms and patterns in your life that may be predominately yin or yang. Consider them when you have read that chapter and add those that will be helpful to your plan.

Conclusion

Here are a few reminders to help you get the most from the visualization exercise you undertook earlier in the chapter. It is important to remember that *we* are the ONLY obstacles in the way of change! It is all too easy to blame outside factors, other people, or to delay and procrastinate. It really is possible to 'be' more flexible. Even if your body does not agree with this statement at present and you have difficulty touching your toes, it is possible to become more flexible within minutes in terms of outlook and attitude.

- Begin to live your dream
- Begin to be who you saw
- Be here now
- Avoid the past (see it as a challenge)
- Be bold, daring and intrepid!
- What have you to lose?
- You are the only obstacle in the way of achieving this dream!

8

Step Three: Setting Off

By now, through diagnosing yourself in the Step One self-assessment section, you will have identified 'where you are' and have a clear picture, through Step Two, of how you would like to re-balance your life. What follows are the tools laid out in two groups within each of the next six sections. Having determined where you need to take a more yin or a more yang approach in the re-balancing programme from the answers you noted down and summarized on p. 123, begin by looking up under the heading(s) of Activity, Stress, Environment, Patterns of Behaviour, Spirit/Chi or Diet and then read any introduction and the 'too yin' or 'too yang' material in the chosen section(s).

Within each there are several practical guidelines, all of them tried and tested and easy to follow. It is important to remember that this re-balancing programme is essentially about making a 'shift' from where your lifestyle or condition appears to be at present. As with steering a boat, you need to push the tiller firmly in the opposite direction! At the same time, be consistent in what you do. If you decide on a programme of physical activity, do it regularly during the ten days rather than give up or change your approach each day. Remember also that any shift in direction will meet with initial resistance. For example, if you do not like getting up early in the morning and you decide that it would make a difference to your life to do that for the ten days, then it will be a challenge and uncomfortable, while your 'old way of being' will encourage you to remain as you were. Or if, for example, you have found relatively yang in many aspects of your health and approach to life at present, you will identify with all the suggestions that I have listed to make you more yang! It is the challenge, the change and the possibility of breaking patterns and stagnation in your life by going in a more yin direction that will make a difference. Left to our own devices, it is always much simpler to invent more of the same.

Fitting these ten days into what may be a busy lifestyle, a distracting lifestyle or social pressures, it is wise to choose a ten-day period when you can give the time and space that you need for yourself. A practical suggestion is to initiate the programme at a weekend and finish the following Monday (ten days later). This gives you time and space at the weekend to initiate changes in whichever area(s) you have chosen to take on. It is also practical if you need to buy ingredients for your diet, organize recreational activity, give yourself time for meditation or begin to examine and bring about alterations within your space at home. It is also far easier, if you give yourself space to deal with any initial 'reactions' to any sudden or radical change.

Remember, if you have identified yourself as being much more yang, to be aware that you are likely to go about this programme more impulsively, quickly, potentially more impatiently – which, if taken excessively, will often lead you to abandon it in impatience. If, however, you have identified that you are more yin then you will need more self-discipline to initiate the programme; be aware of any procrastination on your part and make more effort to avoid being distracted by others or events in your life that could give you the excuse to delay or stop the programme. It is, ultimately, your programme!

ACTIVITY – TOO YIN

If you have decided that you would benefit from taking up a new form of physical activity that is yangizing, here are a few guidelines to help you choose. However, if your current condition is strongly yin and you feel physically out of condition, then although it is important that you start to steer yourself towards yang it is equally important that you do not overdo it. If you are overweight, have high blood pressure or breathing difficulties, always consult a healthcare professional before you set out on any new or challenging exercise programme. Always transition-in slowly but at the same time remember to be consistent. Here are the major factors that I would encourage you to build into your new programme of physical activity:

Warming

Generating heat is a very yangizing process and whatever activity you choose to take up needs to be strenuous enough to get you warm.

Fast

Speed is a yangizing factor so make sure that you build up the pace in whatever you choose to take on. There is little point in undertaking an exercise programme that is very laid-back.

Stimulating/challenging

Not only does the activity need to be physically stimulating and challenging but also mentally. Developing, training, sharpening, challenging our nervous system is just as important in the yangizing process as developing good cardio-vascular power.

Aggressive/competitive

Bringing in some level of competition into what you do is vital. Whether you set yourself a goal that you wish to improve on or whether you participate in a team sport or engage in a racquet sport on a one-to-one basis with your opponent, make sure you go into it with a spirit of giving your best and having the desire to win.

Sweat/breathless

A fundamental guideline, whatever physical activity you choose to undertake, is to make sure that it incorporates the following factors. (Naturally, take into account your age, whether you are overweight or unused to exercise. Do not strain yourself and ask your doctor if you are anxious. Always build up slowly to this level.)

1 You engage in the activity at least four times during this ten-day period.
2 The length of time you participate in your exercise is a minimum of thirty minutes.
3 During your activity you become breathless and begin to break into a sweat. These two considerations show that you are exercising well and you need to judge (or seek advice from a health professional) how long you can endure this pace.
4 Make sure that whatever you undertake is both exciting and challenging. You could fulfil the first three categories simply by running on a treadmill in your local gym. But is it exciting or challenging? Building on a level of excitement or thrill means being able to be spontaneous as you take on the unknown. Many sports and recreational activities can provide you with this element – it is not just about working your lungs and your heart.

Jogging

This is a simple and cost-effective form of exercise that can provide you with a whole spectrum of yangizing qualities depending on how far and how fast you take it on. If you have not jogged for a year or more please make sure that you have the appropriate footwear. Your local sportswear shop can always advise you. Also, always 'limber up' before you leave your home, loosening up your ankles, hips and knees. You can also stretch the backs of your legs by either touching your toes or leaning in at a 45-degree angle towards a wall, applying pressure with the palms of your hands on the wall and bending one of your knees while stretching the back of the other leg. To be very present and focused on what you are doing while you are jogging, leave your portable music system at home! The time and distance of your jog is up to you, but a good half hour three or four times a week is yangizing, daily more so. Pounding the urban streets is far more yangizing – dealing with the traffic, pedestrians and the hard concrete under your feet. Finding an open space such as a beach, parkland, heathland or country lane recharges your Chi in a more uplifting fashion. There is also the added factor in strange country that you have to 'navigate' where you are going. This can bring about greater focus (yang) than running a few circuits near your home. Remember at the end of your jog to unwind by shaking out your wrists, your knees and ankles. Placing the palms of your hands near the sacrum and rotating your hips can also help to loosen and unwind any tight muscles in your back and pelvis.

Good advice if you are not sure about your neighbourhood, or if you have just checked into a hotel and have decided to take a jog, is to ask someone who knows the area the best place to go and also where it is safe. You do not need to have the added yangizing factors of being chased, robbed or mugged as well! Many years ago I stayed with a family outside Nairobi who owned a sizeable property. I was up at the crack of dawn before my hosts and decided to take quick jog before breakfast. I vaguely remember hearing my name being yelled as I quietly shut the back door before setting out and within minutes discovered why. For security reasons, the family had five or six very hungry Alsatian dogs who prowled the property at night to keep any would-be burglars at bay. I had the most yangizing jog of my life as the dogs joined in and I hastily beat a retreat to the back door and pleaded with my hosts to let me in!

Racquet Sports

Sports such as tennis, badminton, table tennis and squash can all bring excellent forms of yang into the game. These qualities include the competitive nature of the sport, the focus and concentration that is required, the need for space and accuracy, the training in agility, and of course the potential for getting breathless and sweaty. It is not too difficult to find a partner who will take you on – it does not require a whole team of you to play. You can put as much pressure into the game as you wish. Tennis and badminton can be taken on at any pace that you desire and have the additional potential to allow you to socialize afterwards which, if you have been feeling more yin and potentially isolated, will also do you good. Table tennis may appear superficially to be a very unchallenging pasttime; however, if played at speed and with a desire to beat your opponent it can be very yangizing. Of all these racquet sports, I find squash the most yangizing of all. Played within the confines of a small court with a relatively small ball and a much smaller racquet than tennis, at great speed and requiring not only agility but foresight – this is yangizing! Don't be too dismayed if your partner has you running around in circles and exhausting you – it's just a symptom that you are still too yin! The intensity, the speed, the pressure and the shortness of the game all contribute to its yangizing effect. Even in half an hour you will find yourself getting breathless and working up a good sweat. It can also be intensely competitive.

Cycling

This is not about taking a leisurely ride on Sunday afternoon along a canal towpath! It is about pushing yourself hard, taking on a challenge route, getting up some speed and bringing in an element of thrill or excitement. If you haven't done any cycling for a while and intend to dust down the old bike sitting in the garage or garden shed then of course make sure that it's in good working order – especially the brakes. Whatever terrain you choose to ride on, it is best to wear the appropriate headgear and make sure that if you are going to ride at dusk or dawn you are visible to other road users. A practical suggestion, if it is appropriate because of time constraints in your life, is to cycle to and from work daily. Of course this has to be practicable in terms of distance, somewhere to leave and lock up your bike, and you don't want to arrive in the office hot and sweaty and in need of a shower five minutes before an important meeting. Cycling can provide you not only with a good source of energetic, physical activity but also help to focus and yangize your nervous system prior to getting to work. The tribulation of the morning rush-hour traffic can potentially give you the edge over fellow workers who have not undergone the same challenges as they commuted in. A cycle ride will leave you invigorated, sharp, focused, awake and alert to what is going to happen next. On the other hand, a leisurely journey into work on public transport in a warm, stuffy, overcrowded bus or train can leave you soporific, tired, uninspired and in a semi-dreamlike state. If you feel the desire and need to become more yang, look at incorporating cycling or another form of exercise that is as challenging before work.

Orienteering

There are clubs and associations all over the world that organize events for people of all ages and abilities. As a recreational activity it is potentially yangizing – not only for your Chi and circulation system but most importantly for your nervous system. If you are not familiar with the sport, you are given a map and compass, various stops or locations that you have to find; and it is up to you to use your skills or map reading and gamesmanship to decide your objectives and the order in which you choose to target them. Most competitors run or jog between the given points, always through unknown territory, at the same time having to bring an almost 'chess-like' approach to the decisions about locations and how to tackle them. You are constantly on the move, always being challenged by the terrain, and your mind is taxed as you decide and implement your plan. Another yangizing factor is that you do this solo – the isolation of the event keeps you focused and reliant only on yourself and your own judgement.

Martial arts

A whole range of different martial arts are available nowadays but essentially they have one common thread. They are designed to help you to be in the moment. Training to be flexible, alert, open and aware of what is going on around you demands a great deal of yang. It is not about aggression or beating people – it is about becoming centred. All martial arts require the discipline of regular practice (yang), a commitment to being on time (yang), training in flexibility, breathing and agility. Some form of martial arts training is now available in almost every major city and town. If you are interested in this approach it is well worth meeting the director, attending an open evening and then enrolling in a beginners' class. The training, the breathing, the discipline and the respect for other students all have a profound 'centring' effect.

Twenty years ago I used to attend Aikido classes two or three times a week for an hour at 7.30 a.m. Making the commitment to be there was yangizing, actually getting there on time, especially deep in the winter, was equally yangizing. The most profound discovery I had from my Aikido practice was how my day began to unfold after a session. The practice session yangized my Chi and as a result I was far more present to my tasks that particular day, and noticed that I was beginning to predict problems before they even arose. On other days, when I had not been to practice, I was far more likely to be on the receiving end of the unpredictable and therefore unprepared. The other insight I developed from this practice was how important it was to avoid aggression and confrontation. The training is not designed to make you look for trouble but to be aware of it and therefore potentially prevent it. Of course, if you should find yourself with your back against the wall, you will have an excellent basis for self-defence.

Challenge programme

Old-fashioned military style and boot camp-like training is becoming more and more popular as a way of yangizing individuals for their work and leadership positions. In recent years middle and top management personnel have shown considerable interest in how to get their people working and co-operating away from the office or the field in which they work. Several companies now offer both to corporate and private individuals the opportunity to enrol in some kind of out-door challenge programme. Many of the leaders and trainers of these have a military background themselves, corporate management skills or some form of group therapy training. It is possible to enrol for a weekend or a week, and if you are lucky to work for a large enough company they may even sponsor you to attend.

Why I believe that this particular approach can be suitably yangizing for a relatively yin person is that there is a structure, a leadership, a group, a challenge and the encouragement and support that are required to make it successful. Often if we are predominantly yin we can lack the motivation to initiate action that could be challenging to ourselves. Another special feature of these courses is that the leaders set out to ensure that it is a win/win situation for all the participants. The yang ones will not get away with rushing off and doing things at their pace oblivious to everybody else's needs and desires, while at the same time the yin ones will be encouraged and supported to see the programme through. From the outset it is clear that it is up to the yang ones to develop patience for the slower people and for the yin ones to increase their pace and contribution, so that eventually both extremes will support each other, meet in the middle and create that universal success. Having been on several of these courses myself, I can only reflect that the experience is profoundly yangizing while giving you the opportunity to share your skills, show your compassion, listen to and respond to the needs of others. If you feel daunted at the prospect, enrol with a friend. But undoubtedly, as the course evolves, that added security will become irrelevant as you merge into the group.

Conclusion

Whatever you choose to take up, whatever you choose to take on, make sure that you are consistent, that you keep your word and that you give it as much effort as you can. When our condition is more yin it really does require a lot of effort to even begin to recognize the value of physical challenge, but it will pay off.

ACTIVITY – TOO YANG

All of us need physical activity and recreation to keep our breathing, our circulation, our Chi and our nervous system in good shape. If you have identified that your current condition is too yang, the following ideas are designed to bring about a more relaxing approach that is more leisurely, quieter and relatively slower.

Yin factors that you could build into your activity could include:

Warmth

Being in an environment that is warm is particularly relaxing, whether this is swimming in a warm ocean, relaxing at a health spa or just keeping well wrapped up when you are out walking or jogging.

Leisurely

Avoid doing things in a hurry or being constrained by some kind of time pressure. There is little point in dashing to your local health spa to squeeze in forty-five minutes of relaxation while you are constantly aware of the time and your next meeting.

Uncompetitive

You may enjoy participating in sports with others and it would be wise for this ten-day period to continue doing so, but minimize any hard-edged competitive quality. Try playing a racket game without scoring for example. A very good way of developing patience is to teach or play or share time in a particular sport with a child. It is good practice for developing patience and sensitivity to their needs as they learn and grow.

Swimming

Provided you can swim, this could prove to be one of the most relaxing and beneficial forms of activity. Make sure that the water is warm, bordering on very warm, and that the atmosphere at the beach or the swimming-pool is geared towards relaxation. Take a good half-hour swim every day during the programme or a minimum of three times a week. Don't adopt a competitive approach: don't count how many lengths or kilometres or time your progress. One of the most relaxing strokes is the breast stroke, which helps to open up the lungs, the chest and, despite any initial stiffness if you haven't swum of a long time, can help release tension in the shoulders and the neck. The important factor here is that the atmosphere should be relaxing. Avoid going to a cold, stark swimming-pool at the crack of dawn, or to an overcrowded complex where it is impossible to relax as you pick a course through screaming and yelling children!

Sailing

This activity has potential for great relaxation – however, it is also potentially extremely yangizing! To make it relaxing you need to make sure that you are very warm, confident and in good company. Ideally choose a day when it is warm and ensure that you do not engage in any competition. Your approach needs to be leisurely and fun. What you don't need is to feel cold, anxious, under pressure or with a friend who turns into a modern-day Captain Bligh the minute he or she steps on to a boat! The fresh air and the moderate challenge create excellent, relaxing recreation.

Fishing

This activity is potentially very relaxing. Plenty of fresh air, a leisurely walk to find a good spot on the bank of the river, an outdoor environment, no distractions and no constraints in terms of time. I personally have found this to be one of the most calming and at the same time energizing forms of activity, whether I go alone, when I am left with my own thoughts and dreams, fish with a friend, or with a child sharing stories and schemes. But fishing is NOT relaxing when you bring in competition. For example, when you count how many fish you have caught, or when you set yourself a time limit, or even try to catch a specific kind of fish. Also to really benefit from the relaxing nature of this activity it is important to keep yourself warm.

Walking

A good long walk in the open countryside at a leisurely pace in good company is undoubtedly one of the best forms of deep relaxation. It is excellent for your circulation, your lungs and being in the open air can re-charge your Chi. It is important that the environment in which you walk is inspiring, that you avoid turning the walk into a route march and that you keep yourself warm. Talking and sharing while you walk and taking regular rest breaks also provide the relaxation that you need. If you are lucky enough to be living in an area that is warm and unpolluted, then to kick off your shoes and walk barefoot on a beach or on a clean path in the woods is very revitalizing and deeply relaxing. Remember that yin Chi rises up through the earth and has a much greater potential to recharge if you have direct contact with the earth rather than being insulated by a heavy pair of boots. Remember how relaxing it was the last time you walked barefoot on a beach or in a meadow.

Children

If you really want to develop a more yin nature one of the most effective ways is to engage in a sport or an outdoor recreational activity with a child. Working at their level, at their pace and from their point of view brings a more leisurely approach and develops patience for you! If you don't have a child or children I am sure that you could borrow one: nieces, nephews, neighbour's child. You could take a cycle ride, play a ball game in the park, go swimming or enjoy a long walk or a racquet sport. The important thing is to make it uncompetitive, fun and let THE CHILD guide the speed of the activity and the approach.

Conclusion

The important factor to bear in mind in inventing and putting into practice any form of physical activity is that there should be an element of fun and that you should make a conscious effort to design something that is essentially very different from your current condition. So having decided that you are relatively yang and need a more yin, relaxing approach, make sure you build it in. The word recreation says it all. It's about re-creating your health and your Chi.

For ten years I led a very pressurized lifestyle in the field of health education and counselling. In addition to this work there was the additional stress of administration, extensive travel and the normal demands of a growing young family. Counselling individuals regarding health-related problems I have always found challenging and exciting. There is an intensity to the work and, because of the need for confidentiality, it is not easy to unwind or share what you have heard or experienced with others. You are sometimes privy to nightmare stories of human suffering and witness all kinds of emotions as well as sharing successes and challenges. In these situations you have to be a good listener, a guide and a coach. Sometimes you need to have a soft, sympathetic approach and at other times to be far more direct and confrontational.

One of my favourite recreational activities during this period of my life was to attend, with my children, at least one a month, a 'demolition derby' at our local speedway stadium! There was a gladiatorial atmosphere in the air; forty battered cars would appear on the track, dust and exhaust fumes in the atmosphere, and a sense of hope that there would be an enormous crash. The children and I loved the action, the spins, the shunts, the wheels coming off; the messier it was the more we cheered and the more we enjoyed it. I began to realize that I was enjoying the carnage, the destruction and the danger. The bigger the crash the bigger the thrill. Having spent most of the week listening to other people's sufferings I was now able to watch others suffer with no feelings of responsibility, but an enormous excitement. Undoubtedly, I was unconsciously releasing pent-up strains from the work. This is a good example of how we need recreation that is fairly extreme to bring about physical and emotional relaxation and release from whatever kind of work and activity that we do.

Soccer spectators all over the world and as far back as the late nineteenth century have enjoyed the potential to release their pent-up emotions through cheering or criticizing the opposite team. For an industrial worker incarcerated in a factory forty to fifty hours a week, living in a confined home in an over-populated industrial city with little chance of travel, holidays or luxury goods, the rewards on a Saturday afternoon of support-ing your team or yelling at the opposition really took the pres-sure off. Even the quiet, sedate and leisurely sport of cricket can stir up the most exuberant emotions in some parts of the world. If you watch a game of cricket in rural England on a Saturday afternoon you will hardly hear a sound. However, witness a game in Calcutta when India are playing and there is a crowd of over 80,000 present. The excitement, the thrill and the release amongst the spectators is awesome.

STRESS – TOO YIN

If your current condition is essentially more yin then you are going to feel uncomfortable in any situation where pressure is brought to bear upon you. Whether this is meeting a deadline, having to make yourself vulnerable or experience greater than normal demands, it will be a very unnerving experience. A yin condition can already manifest as feeling: tired, nervous, pres-surized, overpowered, overstretched or anxious. Put pressure and demands, which are yang factors, on top of this more vul-nerable condition and you will be left feeling low in self-esteem and looking for a way out of the pressure.

Some real physical symptoms can go along with a yin condi-tion faced by yangizing pressures and demands of daily life. These can include: shaking or trembling of the hands and fin-gers, hyperventilation and damp or sweaty palms. Emotionally we can feel trapped, cornered and very vulnerable – eagerly looking for a way to avoid or escape the current pressure. Here are some practical ideas to help you ground your energy, give you focus and clarity while at the same time helping to release some of this excess tension.

Visualization

You have a choice of two exercises here, both designed to bring you qualities of focus, clarity and grounding. As with any visualization exercise, it is important that you follow these guidelines.

1 Find a quiet space where you are guaranteed to be undisturbed for at least ten minutes.
2 Sit (rather than lie down) comfortably with your feet firmly on the floor and your hands relaxed in your lap. Keep your spine as straight as possible.
3 Keep your eyes closed.
4 Relax and breathe from your belly – this will come naturally as you slow down and quieten down your energy.
5 Allow images to come and go without any particular attachment to them.
6 When you are fully relaxed, try one of these two exercises:

The Mountain

Start by bringing forth an image of a mountain. Perhaps it is a mountain you have visited on your travels or it could be an image of one that you have always admired. What is important is that you can feel its presence, its strength, its stability, its security, its majestic and durable nature. Let the image of this mountain fill the whole frame of your vision. Admire it, take its strength and qualities on board as you breathe in. Release your doubts and worries and anxieties as you breathe out. Slowly begin to feel yourself 'become' the mountain. It is important that, if only for a short while, you can identify yourself with its image and its energy. Stay with this visualization as long as it is clear, then when you become restless or the mountain begins to fade, slowly bring yourself back into the present by wriggling your fingers and your toes, stretching and then slowly opening your eyes.

Notice how you feel? Do you feel more grounded? Can you still feel that sense of deep inner security?

Calming the inner storm

Begin by going through the first steps that are outlined in the introduction above and then begin to focus your attention on where you may have physical pain or tension within the body. Use your mind rather like a 'scanning' machine – begin at the top of the head, work your way behind and around your eyes, around the jaw, the neck, shoulders, the chest, the arms and hands, the diaphragm, the abdomen, the pelvis, the legs, the knees, the calves and the feet and toes. As you 'scan' your way down the body be aware of any 'knots' of tension, unusual physical sensations, stiffness or even areas that appear to be under 'anaesthetic'. Choose one of these areas and focus your attention on it. There are two approaches you can take. Firstly, you can release the tension in any given area while you breathe out and make sure that you create an image of dispersion and release. If you are successful in identifying an area of tension, see it leave your body as you breathe out. The out breath provides you with the best platform for freeing the tension.

The second approach to take for disarming an area of tension is to talk to it. This may sound strange, but in the relaxed state that you find yourself in while practising a visualization experience, you have the unique capacity to 'communicate' with the pain, tension and stagnation. Anything is possible at this particular point. The image of another person may come forward. You may just find yourself asking the area what's going on and what it needs. If you are successful in communicating on this level and feel that you get a response that you understand, make it clear to the area that you will take more time in the future to listen to it and to implement what it suggests for changing the situation. A very profound finale to this process of communication is to ask the area for forgiveness – because you have ignored it in the past – and remind it that you will pay more attention in the future.

Keeping your eyes closed and, breathing gently, begin to wriggle your fingers, wriggle your toes and then slowly begin to open the eyes. Try to keep with you the impressions and insights that you gained from the process and keep any promises or commitments that you made.

Physical exercises

Here are four different exercises that you can choose from, all drawn from various oriental bodywork systems and designed to release tension, bring you more focus and to 'ground' you.

1 Drawing the bow

Find a quiet space to be in for 5-10 minutes where you know you will not be disturbed. Preferably have a view in front of you that is open and uncluttered – an open window or, even better, a quiet corner of your nearby park or garden. Next, take off your shoes and release any tension in your ankles and toes by shaking each foot alternately as vigorously as possible. Stand with your feet parallel to each other and with the distance between the feet the same as the width of your hips. Bend your knees very slightly. Keep your back straight, your arms as relaxed as possible and loose by your side and look directly ahead. Try to avoid gazing, daydreaming or staring! Try the old-fashioned Western gunfighters 'snake-eyed' look. Essentially this means narrowing your gaze, relaxing your jaw and looking straight ahead.

Raise both of your arms in front of your body, palms facing down, fingertips relaxed yet outstretched in front of you towards the horizon. Don't let the hands actually touch, keep a distance of at least one hand's width apart. As you breathe in keep your left hand and arm facing straight out in front of you and draw the palm of your right hand over the top of your left hand, wrist, elbow and shoulder (without actually touching the left side at all), still breathing in as you draw your right hand up towards your chin and across your chest; finally, coil up your right arm behind your right shoulder with your palm now facing forward. Hold your breath in this position and, as you breathe out, keep your left arm still outstretched in front of you and gently push your right hand and arm forward with the centre of the palm aiming at the horizon. This first cycle of the exercise is complete when you have completely exhaled and both hands and fingers are facing forward toward the horizon again.

You now repeat the process on the other arm, this time with the right hand outstretched, palm facing down and fingers pointing forward, drawing as you breathe in the left palm across the top of the right hand, wrist, arm and shoulder (about 1 inch/2 cm above the skin) continuing to draw the fingertips of the left hand across the front of your chest underneath your chin, and coiling up the left arm with your palm now facing forward, as far back as you can stretch your shoulder. At this point you hold your breath and as you breathe out repeat the process of slowly pushing your open palm forward until your hand is next to the right hand. Relax the wrist, point the fingers forward and begin to breathe in and repeat on the other side.

You can repeat this exercise 20-30 times and the effect is very calming, grounding and strengthening. The real success lies in your breathing. Try to avoid gushing your breath out as you exhale – it is much better to concentrate and almost assist your breath out as if you were some kind of steam piston. Do it slowly and keep your eyes on the horizon – even if it has to be an imaginary one.

2 The Shake

This is my secret weapon for dealing with butterflies in my belly prior to giving a lecture or appearing on television. Equally you can use this to help calm you down before an interview or before giving that all important presentation. You can practise it anywhere and any time – even at the bus stop.

Stand comfortably with your feet parallel and your feet hip-width apart. Avoid creating any tension in your knees by slightly bending them. Bring your hands behind your back and link your fingertips. There is no need to grip tightly, just a loose linking is quite adequate. Make sure that you are taking long and slow deep breaths, holding them for one or two seconds and then exhaling for at least the same period that you used for inhalation. To complete the exercise, vigorously shaking your intertwined hands up and down behind your back. Three or four minutes of this exercise is enough to placate even the most spirited butter-flies.

What you are doing here is short-circuiting and internalizing your body's natural Chi. Remember that Chi energy moves through meridians that enter and exit the body through the fin-gertips and toes. By short-circuiting this process in the meridi-ans of the upper part of the body you are effectively internalizing this Chi which, coupled with the breathing outlined above, has the effect of grounding and focusing you. Give it a try!

3 The lung stretch

A lot of physical tension that we suffer is caused by poor breath-ing. This next exercise is designed to open the lungs, giving you access to a greater volume of air which in turn helps to calm and alleviate internal stress.

Stand with your feet parallel and hip-width apart. Keep your back straight and look directly out in front of you. Bring your hands behind your back with your arms loose, relaxed and in position just behind the sacrum at the base of your spine. Link your thumbs together and allow your fingers to stretch open. Take a deep breath in and, as you breathe out, bend forward, keeping the backs of your legs straight while at the same time bringing your arms (which remain straight) up as high as you can behind your back. Hold this position until you have fully exhaled and then, as you begin to breathe in, slowly begin to resume a vertical posture and allow your arms to come back (your thumbs remaining linked) behind your back until they are behind the sacrum again. Repeat this exercise 15 times and then repeat the process but this time linking your thumbs the opposite way around.

4 The Cobra

This is a yangizing exercise drawn from the Indian tradition of yoga. Most yoga postures (known as asanas) are generally slow and relaxing. However, with this particular exercise the breathing and posture are made more vigorous and dynamic. Initially, practise the exercise slowly and then build up the pace as your body allows. Obviously the faster you practise this asana the more yangizing the effect will be.

Begin by removing your shoes and any tight or restrictive clothing. Lie face down on the floor on a clean, comfortable mat. Make sure that your legs, feet and ankles are parallel and that the fleshy undersides of the toes are gripping the floor. This means that your ankles will be straight and your Achilles tendons tense. Make sure that your forehead is touching the floor and that you tuck your chin in towards your chest. Keep the muscles around your jaw relatively loose. Finally, place the palms of your hands face down on the floor either side of your shoulders. Now you are ready to begin!

Take a deep, slow inhalation while in this position, hold your breath, then, as you slowly begin to breathe out, push the upper part of your body upwards, raising your head, stretching as far back as possible, Keep your eyes open, keep your hips and pelvis on the floor, keep your toes in contact with the floor and keep the tension in the Achilles tendons. Hold this posture until you have fully exhaled and then, when you are ready, slowly breathe in and lower your chest and forehead to the floor. Repeat this exercise at least 10 times.

Acupressure – Heart-governor no. 8

One of the translations for this traditional acupuncture point is the 'Palace of Anxiety', and it is wonderful for releasing stress, especially tension brought about by anxiety, fear or nervousness. You can easily massage this point on yourself while sitting in a meeting, travelling on public transportation or waiting for the dentist! It is easily found, located at the centre of your palm. The best way to find it is to allow your hand to become loose and relaxed. As the fingers and thumb gently curl inwards, bring the thumb from your other hand across and massage into the hollow at the centre of the palm. It is important to apply pressure while you are breathing out. Rather than stab or prod the point try firmly rotating your thumb into it as you breathe out. Do not apply any pressure while you inhale. Repeat this process at least 20 times on each hand.

Chi Kung – Embracing the oak

This exercise is drawn from the Chinese system of Chi Kung, which is essentially a very dynamic form of 'internal' breathing and meditation that can leave you very centred and grounded. It may appear easy on paper, but it is very challenging, especially the longer you practise it! The exercise allows you to short-circuit your Chi, thereby internalizing it and in this process releasing stagnation and deep stress. As with all Chi Kung exercises the priorities are a) your breathing and b) having your muscles relaxed.

Stand with your feet parallel and a hip's width apart. Have your knee slightly bent, your spine straight, your eyes gazing at the horizon (imaginary or real). Keeping your shoulders relaxed begin by raising your arms in front of you to shoulder height. Imagine that you have directly in front of your body a large oak tree. Loosely 'embrace' this oak by bending your elbows gently, having your palms facing towards your chest and your fingertips aimed tip to tip approximately 2-3 inches (5-7 cm) apart. Try not to let your elbows drop down and be conscious of any ten-sion or stiffness in your shoulders, wrists and fingers. As with all tension-relieving exercises, it is the out breath that provides the link for release. Maintain this posture for as long as you can. It sounds easy but it can be very challenging and uncomfortable.

One of the ways of making this exercise easier is to be aware of any pain and tension and allow it to dissolve with your exha-lation. The minute you start to use muscle the more difficult the exercise becomes. Generally the first few minutes are fine and you begin to wonder what all the fuss is about. Three to six minutes into the exercise you may feel tension building up in your shoulders and chest, a quivering sensation beginning in your wrists and fingers and an overwhelming desire to stop! What is coming up and out is the inner tension. This discharge of tension can last several minutes. Try to ride it out as best you can, allowing all the negativity in your mind to surface and let-ting go of it through your exhalations.

Initially try the exercise for 4 or 5 minutes. Slowly during the 10-day period try to build it up and see if you can achieve 10-15 minutes. This is a very powerful exercise to practise first thing in the morning.

Breathing

The secret to the success of almost every oriental form of body work lies in the art of breathing. At the same time it is true to state that the underlying aggravating factor in physical stress lies in our inability to breath correctly while under stress. One of the most disturbing consequences of poor breathing is hyperventi-lation. Not only are the physical symptoms of feeling dizzy or faint difficult to deal with, but a real sense of panic can set in. A very helpful but symptomatic approach to this problem can be the use of acupressure to stomach point No. 41. This point can be found by tracing the outside edge of your shin bone from your knee towards the top of the foot. Find the area where your foot meets your ankle. Begin by rotating your ankle and feel for the hollow between the tendons on top of the foot precisely where the foot meets the shin bone. Place your thumb in the hollow and apply pressure on the out breath as deeply as possible. Release the pressure as you breathe in and repeat the exercise as you breathe out. Do this at least 15 times on each ankle. If you feel too distressed or too panicky, show a friend or colleague where to press so that you can relax and unwind while the work is done.

The next breathing exercise is designed to release tension and can be practised wherever you are, whether in a meeting, a dentist's chair, travelling on a train or waiting to see your bank manager. Begin by narrowing your eyes so that they are almost closed. Keep your back straight and place your hands in your lap. Preferably have the back of one of your hands gently cupped within the palm of the opposite hand with the thumbs touching. Keeping very still take in a deep breath through your nose lasting 2-3 seconds. Hold this for a further 3 seconds. Now exhale very slowly for approximately 5-8 seconds, but this time through your mouth. Keep your jaw relaxed and your lips only millimetres apart when you breathe out. To really feel the benefit of this breathing exercise, you need to stay with it for at least 3-4 minutes.

Food

If you are feeling yin (vulnerable, worried, anxious, fearful) the last thing that you need to take on board is more yin. The Chi of extremely yin foods and drinks will only add to your feelings of vulnerability and anxiety. To begin with avoid all foods that have sugar in them and any kind of refined carbohydrate. This includes cakes, biscuits, chocolates, pastries and confectionery. Also avoid highly spiced foods which have the capacity to make your 'nervous' Chi more excitable. The strong yin stimulating effect of coffee and commercial teas with caffeine in them will only enhance your tensions and worries.

If when you are feeling nervous and vulnerable at a job interview, your prospective employer offers you coffee and biscuits during the discussion. These stimulating and highly refined yin foods will only fuel your already nervous disposition. Good general advice on food and drink when you are working with yin-related stress is to focus on hot drinks rather than cold; hot meals rather than cold salads; hot desserts instead of frozen ones and always begin a meal with hot soup. Even as a snack, soup can have a very pacifying and calming effect.

Finally, avoid eating too much when you feel you are in a stressful situation. It is far better to eat a comfortable amount of warming foods, chewed very well, than to snack unconsciously while rushing from one commitment to the next. At the same time it is also good advice not to drink too much fluid at this time. This will only stimulate the kidney and bladder energy, increasing your desire to urinate, and when you put the energy of the kidneys under strain you are only adding to your potential to feel fearful and anxious (see Chapter 3).

STRESS – TOO YANG

Many of the physical and emotional symptoms associated with yang-related stress can by symptomatically alleviated by the following methods. Whether we feel physically tight and tense (yang) or emotionally we are irritable, impatient and short-tempered, the process of releasing the stress is much the same. However, it is important to remember that these ideas are only connected with the symptomatic relief of the symptoms and it is important that during the ten-day programme you identify the CAUSE and put into place new ways to help prevent the build-up of stress in the future. It is never easy to advise friends when they are upset to 'calm down', and given that yang's nature is inherently impatient, taking on these exercises will by definition require a lot of time, effort and patience.

Visualization

Before embarking on either of the two visualization exercises, follow the procedure outlined below to get the maximum effect.

1 Find a quiet space where you can be without distraction for at least 10 minutes.
2 Sit in a comfortable chair with your spine erect rather than lying on the floor.
3 Close your eyes.
4 Breathe gently from your belly, noticing the initial shift from your chest to your abdomen.
5 In the initial few minutes allow any images that come to mind to flow in and out of your awareness without becoming attached to them or intellectually involved in questioning what the thought behind them might represent.

The emergence of a butterfly

With your eyes closed bring the image to mind of a chrysalis attached to a branch. Let it fill the whole screen of your imagination. Sense the peace and anticipation of a new beginning. Let your imagination begin to do the work as you see the chrysalis slowly unfurl and the beginnings of a butterfly emerge. Allow your imagination to colour the images of this miracle. Watch as the wings begin to unfurl, how the different colours begin to get brighter within the wings and then take in the sheer beauty and tranquillity of the butterfly. You can also imagine the pressure and effort that was required for the butterfly to break out from its cocoon. Stay with the image for as long as you can, even witnessing its first flight towards freedom. As the image begins to fade or you become distracted by other thoughts, slowly begin to wriggle your fingers and wriggle your toes and finally open your eyes. Notice how you feel. Are you more calm? Are you relaxed? Do you feel less impatient? Are you getting back in touch with the 'big picture' once again?

One of the problems with getting too yang is that you can become too narrow, have tunnel vision and are too caught up in the detail and immediacy of what is going on around you. The purpose of this visualization exercise is to liberate some of the intensity that yang stress inevitably brings.

Releasing the spring

For this exercise, you need to focus your attention on either the heart and chest region or the abdomen. Notice which of these two areas feels more tense. If the physical tension you feel is in your lower back, concentrate on the abdomen; and if the tension you are aware of is in your neck and shoulders then concentrate on the chest.

Bring the image to your mind of a vast, tightly coiled spring. Notice how much tension there is within the coil. Notice if it is getting even tighter. The next step is to place that image within one of the two areas outlined in the paragraph above (chest or abdomen). On the exhalation, start to see the spring gently uncoil. Spend several minutes gently unwinding the coil and releasing the tension on the out breath through the periphery of the body. Pent-up energy in the chest will find a natural release through the meridians of the arms, face and neck. On the out breath see the tension dissipate and leave the body via one of these routes. Yang tension caught up in the belly will find an easier path through the meridian of the legs which exit through the soles of the feet and the toes. Encourage the release of tension on the out breath by this route. Take as long as you want with this exercise and when you feel more relaxed or distracted or the image begins to fade, slowly begin to wriggle your fingers and toes and slowly open your eyes. Notice if your breathing has become deeper and slower. Do you have a more relaxed perspective on the task in hand? Can you see different ways of approaching your work?

Physical exercises

Here are four practical exercises designed to help you release bottled-up stress. As with all forms of body work, the breathing is the key to success. However, in this instance because the inner stress is of a more yang nature, it is important that your breathing is bold and even vociferous on the exhalation! This can include: grunting, shouting or releasing the tension with a large sigh.

1 Tarzan

This is a wonderful exercise for releasing tension in the chest-lung-and-heart meridian. Stand with your feet parallel and hip-width apart; relax your knees by keeping them slightly bent; gaze ahead towards the horizon and have your hands loose by your sides. As you breathe in, come up on to your toes and stretch your open hands above and out to the sides of your head at 45° to your shoulders. You can also lean or tip your head slightly backwards at the same time. Gaze upwards while you are in this posture. Hold your breath for a second and clench your fists. As you breathe out bring your heels back to the ground and begin to pound with loose wrists on to the area just below your clavicle on either side of your neck. While pounding and breathing out bring in the extra dimension of release by incorporating a loud, vigorous Tarzan call! Repeat the exercise 4 or 5 times.

The lung meridian and heart meridian can both be found on the inside soft part of the arms. The initial stretch opens up the meridian while the exhalation process and the pounding help to release built-up tension within these two systems. It is a very effective exercise when we have become too tight (yang).

2 Releasing the yang

There are all sorts of tricks of the trade for releasing a very tight nut on a bolt in engineering or for undoing a tight lid on a bottle or jar at home. There are gadgets, gizmos and loosening oil. However, there is also an old yin/yang technique that we have all employed. If something is too tight it is obviously too yang. We are trying to release – yinize – it. Yang, taken to its extreme, will turn into its opposite. One of the simplest solutions to undoing a nut or a lid that is too tight, is to tighten it up even further! This is the logic behind this neat exercise.

Stand with your feet parallel and hip-width apart, with your knees slightly bent. Gaze ahead towards the horizon. As you breathe in tense up your fists, wrists, forearms, shoulders, neck and even screw up the muscles of the face and the eyes. Hold this tension like a coiled spring. Even quiver with the tension. When you can no longer take the pressure, release with a short and loud out breath – allowing all the tension to disappear from your face, neck, shoulders, arms, wrists and hands. Repeat the exercise 3 or 4 more times. The tighter you wind yourself up the more capacity you have to unwind in the opposite direction.

3 The dog shake

One of the most effective releases of tension and one that we have a natural ability to tap into is spontaneous movement. We are doing it all the time. Whether this is yawning or stretching, rubbing or scratching – these are all subtle releases or stimulations that we unconsciously employ. The most active time for this so-called spontaneous movement is during sleep. The way we lie, the way we stretch, the way we breathe all help release and recharge our body.

For this exercise you need to imitate the actions of an excited and playful dog. Imagine such a pet who has been released from the confines of its owner's home after hours of incarceration. The dog will run around madly, chase everything in sight, be exuberant, over playful and will enjoy rolling and lying on its back. It's amazing to watch a dog in the park release this pent-up tension in such a way. Now you need to do much the same! Make sure you are wearing loose, comfortable clothing and begin by lying on the floor. Raise your legs and your arms so that the palms of your hands and the soles of your feet are facing the ceiling. Begin by shaking your ankles and your wrists as vigorously as you can while at the same time making as much noise as you wish! The shaking process releases the pent-up Chi within the body, whereas the free-spirited expression helps to release knotted up emotions.

4 Yoga stretch

This is a powerful exercise that is best used either a) at the end of a long stressful day when you want to completely unwind or b) if you have insomnia because either your mind is too active (yang) or your body is too tense (yang).

Make sure that you are wearing loose, comfortable clothing and avoid doing this exercise on a soft mattress – it is much better to use the floor provided you are warm and there is some kind of basic cushioning. Begin by lying on your back and have your feet together and your arms relaxed by your side with your fingers pointing down towards your toes. Bring your chin in towards your chest and make sure that your jaw is relaxed. Begin by stretching the Achilles' tendons – this can be done by pointing your toes towards your face. Keep the tension on during the exercise. Next, raise your forearms, keeping your elbows tucked in by your sides and your palms facing up towards the ceiling. You are aiming to arch your back by raising your belly and lower back off the floor while supporting yourself on your heels, upper arms and elbows. Breathe in, keep your chin close to your chest and have maximum tension within the body as you hold the inhalation in this arched 'brute-like' posture. Hold the position for as long as you can – 2-10 seconds – and then release quickly. This means that you let go of all the tension in your neck, shoulders, arms and ankles, allowing the body to flop quickly and spontaneously back to the floor while you breathe out in one short breath. You only need to practise this three times. Then relax and gently rock your hips from side to side for half a minute.

The release of tension during this exercise is enormous. However, do not overdo it. Two to three times is quite adequate. Do not attempt this exercise if you have any lower back or neck problems.

Acupressure – Gall-bladder no. 30

One of the side-effects of becoming too yang in stressful situations is that we can becomes increasingly intolerant, impatient and hypersensitive on a sensory level. This means that we become irritated by draughts, noises, smells and even touch. The organ in oriental medicine that controls our patience and sensitivity to the outside world is the gall-bladder. Massaging this point can symptomatically bring about relief by helping to discharge some of this pent-up energy. The gall-bladder meridian and its Chi also play a vital part in our capacity to develop patience and planning. However, when we are too yang the gall-bladder Chi goes into overdrive facility. This makes it very difficult for us to relax or be in the moment. As a result we feel constantly under pressure, irritable and are always thinking about what to do next.

Gall-bladder no. 30 is located in the hollow found on the cheek of the buttocks. Begin by placing your hand on your hip and then allow your fingers to slide down the front of the pelvis. Your thumb will now be in the region of the 'dimple' at the side of the buttocks. This is the hollow where gall-bladder 30 is located. Press as hard as you can into the point as you breathe out and then lean your body against the pressure. For example, if you begin with the left side, locate the point with your left thumb on the left buttock, breathe in and, as you breathe out, bend your hips towards the right, push your thumb deeply towards the right while at the same time leaning your torso and head toward the left. Repeat on the other side, completing both sides at least six times.

Tai Chi

One of the challenges of dealing with yang-related stress is how to tame or channel that internal tension. You can't tell it to go away. Staring at a blank wall in meditation will probably make you even more tense. But imagine a system of moving meditation that allowed you freedom of movement and freedom of breathing, both essentially yin qualities. Tai Chi is increasingly popular in the West and what I introduce here is simply a warm-up exercise that might precede any Tai Chi class.

Begin by standing with your feet parallel and hip-width apart. Keep your knees loose and slightly bent. Stare out into the middle distance and make sure there is no tension in your jaw. Let your arms hang loosely by your sides. Keeping your gaze ahead of you begin by turning your hips and shoulders gently from side to side. While doing this bend your knees slightly as you turn fully to the right or fully to the left. Now bring your arms into play. As you swing your hips gently towards the right allow your right arm to swing around loosely in front of your body, slapping your left hip while your left arm swings behind, the back of your left hand almost touching the top of your right buttock.

Keep up this gently swinging motion, bending your knees and allowing your arms to get involved. Try not to make anything happen. Do not use any muscle in your shoulders, wrists or forearms. Soon you will find the movement builds into a natural flowing meditation.

With practice you may want to bring in a different style to how you place your feet and ankles. For example, as you swing to the left, keep your right foot firmly placed on the floor with your toes pointing out in front of you, but pivot on your left heel bringing your toes high off the ground until your foot faces 90° to the left. Then, as you swing to the right, bring your left foot to face forward and swivel your right foot on your heel with a good stretch of your Achilles tendons as your toes point up. I suggest you do not attempt to bring this level in until you have got used to the swinging and breathing first.

Breathing

This is undoubtedly the simplest approach to dealing with yang-related stress. Whenever you find yourself getting tense notice how you are breathing. Even in a tense meeting it is possible to take time out to be aware of this and to follow the routine described below. You only have to witness the incredibly yang-gizing process of giving birth to realize how important breathing is. It is as if the body goes into automatic to deal with the massive load of stress and tension that is involved.

Sitting very still with your shoulders relaxed and your hands in your lap, begin by being aware that you are breathing in and out through your nose. It is important that your breathing is deep, slow and quiet. You can check the depth of your breathing by noticing whether your abdomen contracts and expands on the inhalation. Make the in breath through your nose approximately 3-4 seconds, do not hold your breath and then make the exhalation between 6-8 seconds in duration. The releasing quality of this form of breathing is based on the softness of your breath. If you were to hold a piece of light tissue in front of your nostrils, the power of your exhalation would not even cause it to ripple. If it is appropriate at the time, close your eyes as you practise this breathing. Three to five minutes is an adequate period to feel the calming effect.

Food

When we feel under stress with the additional factor that we are already too yang, then we are most likely to do things quickly, impetuously and in a restless manner. Avoid building on this way of being by eating too quickly, rushing around while you eat, talking, having a telephone conversation or reading a report. It is vital that when you eat you chew very, very well. Realistically, try to make this thirty or more times per mouthful. Put your eating implement down between each mouthful and chew until whatever you are eating becomes liquid.

It would also be wise to avoid at this time foods that have more yangizing effect on your condition. Avoiding food that is overcooked; reduce your use of baked products – pies, pastries and toast; never add salt or soya sauce to your food at the table; avoid reheating food as this makes it even more yang. There are also certain categories of food that are extremely yang – namely smoked salmon and tuna. If you are scanning the sandwich bar for a pleasant relaxing lunch when you are too yang, the worst thing you could pick up would be a tuna or smoked salmon sandwich!

There are plenty of relaxing herbal teas on the market and you would undoubtedly benefit from the mild, soothing effect of camomile tea rather than the stimulating effect of coffee. Although essentially coffee is a yin product, it has a tendency to exaggerate or enhance the quality of Chi that you already have – whether it is excessively yin or yang.

Warm drinks, fresh vegetables, salads, pasta, rice and local seasonal fresh fruit all have a gently relaxing and calming effect. On a more subtle level, the more natural, gentle energy of a gas flame is infinitely better than the pressurized sporadic nature of microwave energy, which you would be wise to avoid when you feel under yang stress.

ENVIRONMENT

As an art or as a science, Feng Shui could fill a book with its principles and practice. However, there are some fundamental features to this ancient Chinese art, based on yin/yang thinking, that have the potential to benefit your Chi and well-being. Given that you spend at least half your life at home and up to one-third of a day asleep, then it is vitally important to realize that your home not only mirrors how you feel but has the potential to recharge or even drain you. The following ideas are drawn from different schools of Feng Shui and can provide you with simple and common-sense suggestions for bringing about change within your space.

Clutter and disorder

Have a very good look at your space for a moment. Does it give you the impression of tidiness or disorder. It is no good hiding all the clutter in those bedroom cupboards either! Take a look outside – whether it is the area around your front door or the space that you may have at the back of the property.

Remove all sweet wrappers, leaf debris, broken plant pots, unwanted junk mail, and dead plants from the vicinity of your front entrance.

Find a suitable place to store your dustbin so that it does not sit outside your front door.

Distinguish clutter. A good definition is items within your space that you rarely use. These could include: old letters; a large collection of sentimental memorabilia; projects that realistically you are unlikely to complete; stuff that belongs to friends or relatives that you are storing for them; clothes you have grown out of; old accounts; chequebook stubs that you no longer need to keep. You need to go through all this and ruthlessly get rid of what is not absolutely necessary. Winter clothing, sports equipment and holiday clothing that you are not currently using is not technically clutter but needs to be stored out of the way at present. Having a clutter-free zone at home has the benefit of a) keeping your mind clear and b) allowing new possibilities to enter your life.

Entrances

The opening into your home is vitally important as it is symbolic of the entrance of Chi (life force) into your space. Make sure that you keep the entrance way free for the traffic of people and Chi – find another place to store the bicycle! It is essential to keep your doormat clean and regularly vacuumed, shake or replace it. Make sure that the entrance way feels welcoming – no glaring lights – while at the same time it creates an atmosphere that is warm, cheerful and welcoming. This can be achieved by fresh flowers and paintings that give any visitors a sense of calmness.

Repairs

Take a note pad and wander around your space making a note of everything that needs attention. It is vital that you do this exercise as objectively as possible. Particular areas to pay attention to include: taps that drip; doors that squeak; panes of glass or light bulbs that need replacing; a clock that keeps irregular time; a door bell that does not function; a stain on the carpet; a broken drawer; any fuses that need replacing; drains that are blocked or that have potential to block in heavy rain. When we live with these small malfunctions all the time, we constantly unconsciously remind ourselves that we must do something about them. For example, you could open the refrigerator where the light bulb has not been working for the past six weeks. You have completely got used to the fact that it is not functional but on a subconscious level you notice it, it distracts and annoys you. Once you have made your list, declare when and how you are going to get the jobs done! The living environment that works smoothly will begin to rub off on you in terms of relaxation and will be mirrored in other areas of your life that will begin to work more effortlessly.

Your bedroom

This space is fundamental to your well-being. We spend up to a third of our life asleep and during this process we are naturally deeply relaxed (yin) while we regenerate ourselves for the next day. It is therefore vital that this space is peaceful and that you feel secure within it.

No busy-ness

Keep all the trappings of your working life out of this space as much as possible. Do not leave your mobile phone to re-charge in the bedroom. Certainly do not keep your fax machine or personal computer in this area. If, for pressure of space, you have a bureau or a desk that you work at for a portion of the day, make sure that you can stow it away or 'hide it' with a screen or a drape. The yangizing influence of work-related activities does not engender a feeling of peacefulness.

Colours

Avoid very bright colours such as pure white or red or predominately dark colours such as black. Shades of blue and yellow, orange and mauve have a more restful quality. Red is symbolic of passion and if you wish to embrace more of this in your life you can introduce small areas of the colour: a red lampshade, a touch of red on the curtains or the bedspread, or certain wall fixtures that are red. Obviously avoid red carpets, red wallpaper, red curtains and red bedspreads – too much is potentially overbearing!

Mirrors

While mirrors can be used wisely to open up your space or enhance areas that appear dark or gloomy, they can equally drain your energy while you are asleep. If you lie on your bed notice if you can see your image in a mirror anywhere in the room. If you can then you need to remove or cover the mirror. While you are in a vulnerable yin state asleep, the mirror is draining your Chi. If you need a full-length mirror to dress by, try hanging it on the inside of your wardrobe instead.

A sense of security

Subconsciously, we all feel the desire to feel safe in whatever space we occupy. Have you noticed that when you take a seat in a restaurant or train you feel far more comfortable if you can see the door. The same is true when you are asleep. Subconsciously, you will feel more relaxed and more at ease if you can see the door from the position of your bed.

Stability

Another quality to bring into your bedroom that will help you deeply relax is to have a good support behind your head. This means avoid sleeping with your head up against a window or a radiator. The best advice is to ensure that you have a solid structure behind your head in the shape of a headboard. Ideally this is made of wood; it can be covered with soft material if you wish, but it needs to be solid. Bars and latticework headboards do not provide you with the same 'support'.

Clutter

Keep this room absolutely clutter-free. By all means have a laundry basket but do not leave your clothing and shoes in untidy piles. Check the area for old magazines, books and notes that are gathering dust. Make sure also that there is a clear route to and from your bed and to any cupboards and doors that you may use. Ideally the routes that you take should be unimpeded by too much furniture and especially clutter.

Sharp edges

Furniture, fixtures and fittings in your bedroom should have rounded and smooth surfaces. Avoid bedside tables, cupboards and shelving units with sharp edges. The corners of these types of furniture direct negative energy out from the 90° angle that they create. Check the area close to your bed and make sure that you are not in the 'firing line' of any of this negative Chi. Being on the receiving end of this kind of Chi can leave you feeling attacked, uncomfortable and insecure. It can even manifest in low grade ache and pains within your body, particularly the area at which these cutting edges are aimed at.

Images

What you wake up to in the morning is symbolic of how you will view the day. Looking out at a blank wall or a dark cupboard or a chest of drawers covered in files, is not exactly inspiring. Ideally, select a painting, a poster or a piece of art work that inspires you. This could be an image of somewhere that you have been from which you gained great inspiration. It could be symbolic of growth, the dawn, or warmth. Hang this image opposite your bed so that upon waking it is the first impression you receive, whether this is consciously taken in or subconsciously experienced. Make it as big as you can!

ENVIRONMENT – TOO YIN

A very large open space can leave you with feelings of emptiness, loneliness or coldness, all yin factors. If you are feeling uncomfortable because of the size of a particular room, start to bring in more yang factors. These might include softer lighting, more heating, warm coloured carpets (shades of reds and yellows); and you can soften the expanses of walls with tapestries and other soft furnishings; soft screens and full curtains can also help to break up the space in a gentle way.

Too dark

Check areas of your home where it feels particularly gloomy. Look at what you can do to improve the lighting. Uplighters strategically placed in dark corners can begin to open up your space. If you have a hallway that receives very little natural light use long-lasting low wattage light bulbs that can be left on all day without burning too much power.

Multifaceted crystals have the capacity to bring in light and Chi. These are best hung inside a window approximately 15° above your eyeline. Whatever daylight these crystals receive they will multiply and radiate into your space. But remember that because they have the capacity to enhance what they receive and reflect into your space, the crystals will inevitably enhance any negative influence outside the window. This could be your neighbours' washing line or a tall imposing building. In these cases they are best avoided.

Too old

Old buildings have a special Chi of their own and the positive attributes can include a feeling of stillness, restfulness and reflection. Some negative attributes are stagnation, isolation and feeling blocked. It is vital that you keep the space very clean and functional. Try not to live in a space that is in great need of repair or to surround yourself with objects that are broken or no longer work. All of this will rub off on your progress, slowing you down, inhibiting your potential for change and constantly distracting you.

Damp

It is vital for your health that you discover the cause of any dampness and go to whatever lengths are needed to deal with it. Symptomatically you can use a de-humidifier during the day when you are out. Get advice regarding your heating system and make sure that you have adequate ventilation as the circulation of air, rather like Chi, is essential for ensuring that this yin stagnant quality does not occupy your space.

Plants

Healthy plants can bring a bright, fresh charge into your space. Avoid having bunches of dried flowers, pot pourri or stale cut flowers in your home. Plants, like us, need sunlight, air and good Chi. I particularly like ferns as they require plenty of attention from the owner. Use them to brighten up your space as well as being a good barometer of your current health.

Electric/microwave cooking

One of the turning points in our evolution as human beings was discovering and harnessing fire. Once we began to cook our food the process of communication, cultivation and primitive industrial activity began. What is a flame? It is a microcosm of the sun. The sun gives us life as we know it, vitality, Chi and all the manifestations in our natural world. It has only been in the last hundred years that we have begun to experiment with new types of flame. Undoubtedly, electric and microwave cooking has a yinizing effect on both our food and our Chi. The practical solution is to use a 'flame' in our daily cooking (gas).

Feeling isolated

One of the most powerful ways to regenerate the Chi in your home is to host a party. Not a quiet dinner party for three or four old friends but a party party! Plenty of food, drink, music and Chi. Undoubtedly throwing a party disturbs and distracts the Chi of your home. When your guests have a great time and bring with them their laughter and boisterousness it will all rub off on your space. Long after they have gone and you have cleaned up and dealt with all the breakages, you will feel that there has been a shift in the Chi of your home. Provided everyone had a great time, it can only enhance your feelings of warmth and companionship.

Unmotivated

Bring images of activity into your space. These could be scenes from nature of high winds or crashing waves. They could be images of sport or of success - perhaps a famous poster of a sporting hero receiving acclaim. What you don't need are pictures of stagnant lakes, sunsets, graveyards or other symbols of the past.

Music can bring a whole new vibration on a Chi level to your home. Select something that uplifts your Chi and keep it fairly loud.

Bring a new fresh fragrance into your space using an essential oil burner. Fill the small reservoir at the top with water and add four or five drops of rosemary essential oil. Heat the reservoir with a small night light and the aroma of rosemary will begin to pervade your space. It has a very stimulating and penetrating quality which can help deal with indecisiveness, tiredness or lack of memory or motivation.

ENVIRONMENT – TOO YANG

If you feel that the walls are closing in on you and it is impractical to expand, you can 'open up' your space by using mirrors. The shiny glass surface has the power to enhance a particular area or give it a feeling of space. But it is important to remember that a mirror will exaggerate whatever it is facing. If your space is untidy and disorganized then a strategically placed mirror will only give you more of the same.

Make sure that your mirror is clean. It is far more beneficial to reflect a bright, sharp image. Check it for any hairline cracks as these have the possibility of 'distracting' your energy. Broken images reflected into your space are also capable of creating broken or 'scatty' energy. It is therefore wise to avoid the type of mirrors that are used for tiling.

Too bright

Bright lights and strong sunshine have a powerful yangizing effect. Just remember what it feels like to have your bedroom light turned on in the middle of the night – confronting, uncomfortable and very disquieting. Bamboo or venetian blinds are a pleasant way of breaking up harsh sunlight and dimmer switches and soft glow light bulbs can help reduce the harshness in most lighting systems. The worst kind of lighting is undoubtedly fluorescent – which by its nature can leave us feeling agitated and hyperactive – a little bit like what is going on inside the fluorescent tube.

Too hot

Excessive heat as with excessive pressure creates a yangizing effect. Make sure that you have a good circulation of air and if excessive heat is a constant problem because of the climate in which you live, look at the use of cooling colours on your walls and within your soft furnishings. But whatever the temptation, please try to avoid air-conditioning. It can give you a false sense of a change in season while at the same time the cooling effect can divorce you from the reality of the world in which you live. Prolonged use of air-conditioning in a hot climate can leave you out of touch with your environment, your neighbours and the larger community.

Modern

Fashions come and go regarding home furniture but very cold, sharp, clinical almost office-style furniture always has a yangizing effect upon your Chi. It is ideal for the workplace where you need focus and clarity, but it is hardly relaxing. While there is a lot to be admired in a minimalist or Yen living space, it is important to remember that it is essentially yang and you need to bring in the 'yin'. This could be by way of toning down too much grey or white within the colours and looking at practical ways to soften the sharp edges on the furniture. For example, you could drape tablecloths over sharp-edged pieces of furniture, or place plants that have a tendency to grow downwards to mask the sharp edges as they project into the room.

Dry and arid

You can change the atmosphere in the room by introducing a simple form of humidification. This could be a saucer of water placed on a radiator with five to ten drops of pine essential oil. This oil has been traditionally used as a decongestant – opening up and yinizing the airways of the throat and the head.

Computers

The speed, power and activity of personal computers are essentially yang, and if they take up a lot of your domestic space then naturally their energy will pervade your home. It is not a good idea to use or keep your PC within your sleeping space as the activity that the PC generates also has the potential to disturb your sleep. However, some of the negativity that is emitted by PCs can be absorbed by a chunk of either rose quartz or amethyst placed above the terminal.

If you work from home, then once you have declared your work day over consciously shut down the PC. Essentially this means covering it, stowing it or placing a screen around it. Do not allow its presence to dominate your relaxation and recreational time.

Too busy

When your energy is frenetic, speedy and frequently distracted, you need to look at ways of stabilizing and grounding your Chi. Objects that are symbolic of this stability are rocks, stones, pebbles, statues, bronzes. If you feel you are always rushing in and out of the door, place one of these heavier objects near the door to ground you. If you have a staircase that sweeps down towards your front door and you find yourself spending more time out of the house with numerous distractions, place the symbolic heavier item at the base of the stairs to slow down this flow.

Are you finding that you are busy and distracted to the point where you are missing out on opportunities. If this is happening check whether the Chi is flowing excessively out of your home. A good example of this is when you have a window or a door opposite your main front door. Then whenever you open the front door Chi is either rushing in or rushing out – as with any draught created by a simultaneously open front and back door. To slow down this excessive force of Chi place a wind chime in the direct flow. Hang it high enough so that you don't keep banging your head but low enough to be in line with the 'draught' of Chi.

Cannot relax

A subtle way to change the Chi of your space to make it more yin and thereby more relaxing would be to use the vibrational qualities of sound and aroma. Music can provide a relaxing edge to your environment provided it is not too loud. Background sounds of the sea are also subconsciously deeply relaxing.

In addition you could buy an essential oil burner and fill the reservoir with water, heat this up with the flame of a small night light and add five or six drops of lavender essential oil. Traditionally, lavender helps to bring about relaxation and release hyperactivity, fears, worries, irritability and impatience.

PATTERNS OF BEHAVIOUR – TOO YIN

It would be superficial to claim that you could change the habits of a lifetime in a ten-day period. However, as with all the other recommendations in this book, you can become aware of your position and begin to make the effort to swing the pendulum in the opposite direction. The yin patterns are essentially centred on our loss of confidence, feelings of being a victim and are where creativity and self-expression can be stunted by low esteem. The ideas that follow are designed to begin to swing these patterns in an opposite direction by emphasizing strengths rather than weaknesses.

Visualization

This particular exercise is designed to help you dissolve any fear or criticism that has been aimed at you in your life and that you judge could be the cause of any tendency to feel yourself a victim. During the exercise you will be invited to think of a person that has knocked your self-confidence in the past and forgive them. It sounds simple but is extremely effective. Good advice when you practise this visualization exercise for the first time, is to think of a person in your recent past who has upset you. It could be quite a trivial instance at work or with a neighbour. (I wouldn't go for important incidents to do with, for example, one's parents or previous partner without the help of a guide or therapist to help you deal with what comes up.)

Find a quiet space where you will be undisturbed for at least 15 minutes. Sit comfortably with your back straight, close your eyes and keep your body completely relaxed. Make sure that even the muscles in your jaw are relaxed - even if this leaves your mouth feeling loose. Breathe from your belly and allow any thoughts to come and go without getting attached to them. When you feel ready, imagine yourself in a room that is sparsely and simply furnished. See yourself sitting in a chair with an empty chair opposite. Somewhere in the room there is a door. Now think of a person that has been critical of you recently or who intimidated you or knocked your self-confidence. Allow the image of that person to come to mind. Notice how you feel about them. The next step is for you to see them enter the room, greet you and sit in the chair nearby. Make eye contact with them and notice how you feel. Here is the challenging part of the exercise – forgive them! This is the world of fantasy and visualization which gives you the freedom to be who you like. Notice how you feel and how their expression changes when you forgive them. As you direct your thoughts of forgiveness towards them, feel the release of tension in your heart and in your breathing. Be with this release of emotion, the feeling of compassion that you now have, as it will help any resentments that have built up to dissolve.

As the image or the exercise begins to lose power, it is time to say farewell. You can do this in whatever manner seems appropriate. It could be a big hug, it could be a handshake – but whatever farewell you give them it needs to be honest, open and forgiving. See them leave the room and be with how you feel for a few minutes before slowly opening your eyes. The first time I practised this exercise, the person I forgave rang me completely by surprise that evening and we had the most stimulating conversation. Changing my vibrational attitude towards them had given me a new opportunity to communicate. Instead of being defensive, I was relaxed. On reflection, I wondered if there had ever really been a problem or if it had simply been my interpretation of the initial conversation which had impacted on preconceived ideas.

Mirror exercise

Having a negative self-image can really undermine your confidence. Find a large mirror in your home, perhaps at a dressing table, and sit comfortably in front of it. Relax the muscles in your neck and shoulders and spend 4 or 5 minutes daily just looking at yourself. At first you may find you are even more critical of yourself and want to hide. Ride through these negative thoughts until you begin to pick up on what is positive about yourself. It does not have to be 'how' you look but more your presence. Breathe out any negativity that you feel and breathe in the qualities that you admire in yourself or the qualities that you wish to strengthen.

You are a star

Take a few minutes of your time to draw up a chronological list of events in your life where you consider yourself successful. These successes are not necessarily the kinds of accomplishment that others would recognize, but ones that you feel deeply proud of. As you draw up this list you will find that several events have occurred that you have not even begun to acknowledge. Do not include any that have any implications of difficulty or suffering. Here are some examples you might list:

- You came through a challenging birth

- You began to walk at a younger age than your siblings
- You learnt to swim when you were very young
- You were a big hit in your school nativity play
- You won a prize at school
- You paid for your first car
- You were short-listed for an important job interview
- You cancelled a holiday to take care of a sick relative or friend

Go through the list several more times and include even small events where you felt proud and believed that you had accomplished something even if it was not recognized. Later, you can tidy up the list, type it to provide you with a clear presentation of what you have fulfilled. This list is private and you can read it on a daily basis during the ten-day programme to acknowledge what you have achieved and to realize what you are capable of.

PATTERNS OF BEHAVIOUR – TOO YANG

When our overall condition becomes too yang for too long, we can become very impatient, prejudicial, inflexible, arrogant or selfish. Given that the nature of yin and yang is that at their extremes they will begin to turn into their opposites, it is important to remind ourselves that life is not all one-way traffic. The more yang we become the more likely we are to swing the other way, becoming vulnerable, anxious or even doubting our own abilities. To help offset any violent and uncomfortable swings in the opposite direction, these exercises can make that shift more gentle.

Visualization

This exercise is designed to help dissolve any aggression, insensitivity or inflexibility that you may have displayed to someone recently. You are invited to call to mind an individual who you may have upset recently by any selfish or forceful communication you have had with them.

Find a quiet space where you can be undisturbed for at least 15 minutes. Sit in a comfortable chair with your eyes closed, bringing your breathing into your abdomen and allowing all the tension to disappear from your neck and shoulders, eyes and jaw as you breathe out. When you feel 'present' to the exercise, see yourself in a field, a meadow or a wood that you have visited. It needs to be a special place that has relaxing and special memories for you. See yourself in this space sitting comfortably and at one with the world. Coming into view is someone that you are aware you have upset recently. Greet them warmly, see them sit down next to you and maintain eye contact with them. Ask them for their forgiveness. Apologize for your behaviour. Point out that that is not who you really are. Notice how you begin to feel during the exercise and see the new friendship and love that they communicate to you through their eyes. When the image begins to fade, acknowledge them again, give them a big hug and see them wander off towards the horizon. Stay with the feeling of relaxation and release that the exercise brings. Slowly begin to wriggle your toes and your fingers and begin to open your eyes.

The mirror

Spend a few minutes daily sitting comfortably in front of a large mirror at home. Take a good look at yourself and breathe in your strengths, your positive nature and breathe out what you see or feel as a criticism of yourself. Use your imagination to help you see yourself becoming more soft, gentle, open and flexible. Tune into the area of the mouth, the lips and the eyes. See them become softer. This is a very confronting exercise and you need to ride through the initial apprehension and discomfort that it may cause. Try to do this exercise every day during the ten-day programme.

Dissolving exclusivity

There is a tendency, when we become too yang, for us to believe that we are right all the time, that we know better, that ours is the best opinion, that everybody else is too slow, that our intellect is the sharpest. Enormous pressure at work along with the short-term successes that can result, can contribute to this way of being. The more intensely yang we become the more difficult it is for us to see either a bigger picture of what is going on or to hear the ideas of others. The exercise here may then seem to be a nightmare.

a) Take time every day to read a tabloid newspaper from cover to cover! Don't just read the headlines or the articles that may mildly interest you – read everything including the problem pages, the sports pages and the letters. Cover to cover means cover to cover! Remember that this is how a vast majority of the people in your culture hear about and read about the world in which we live. Tune into what they are being made aware of.

b) On three evenings during the ten-day programme watch a minimum of two hours of prime time television – non-stop. Again, before you throw away this suggestion in horror, remember that millions of people around you, people who you share the world with, will be watching this kind of television. This is not designed to be some kind of mental torture but an exercise to help tune you in to how the people around you see and experience the world.

Years ago, I undertook some coaching to help me improve my skills of communication in both counselling and lecturing. My coach asked me what my dream was? I answered that it was to communicate self-healing ideas to as many people as possible. I was given these two tasks to do over a one-week period and defiantly refused to do them. My logic was that I simply didn't have the time to watch prime time television and I certainly didn't want my mind cluttered up with tabloid journalism. My coach pointed out that since at least 75 per cent of my 'neighbours' in the world watched and read and were influenced by these forms of media, if I wished to communicate with them I needed to understand what they read and listened to. My 'punishment' was to be given two papers a day and 4 hours of TV! Looking back, it really helped me to dissolve any exclusive attitude about what I had to offer, how it was different, was better, had more depth. Give it a try!

CHI/SPIRIT – TOO YIN

When our Chi becomes too yin, it can make us naturally over-cautious, tired, out of touch and in need of more sleep and our own space. Shifting this in an opposite (more yang) way will require some initial effort. Here are some lifestyle ideas to help initiate this swing:

Surprise yourself daily

For this ten-day programme do something spontaneous every day to which you would normally be unattracted. Instead of holding back in an argument or confrontation, try taking a stand, make yourself heard and have people listen to you views or opinions. Commit yourself to doing something that normally you would avoid. It could be a project at work that requires more attention or it could be accepting an invitation to dinner that you would normally decline.

Make an effort to socialize more if your overall Chi has for many months been too yin and you have found yourself increasingly isolated, avoiding making commitments and consistently turning down invitations to parties or the movies. It is time to turn this around and for you to initiate the invitation. At first it will take a little bit of work because people around you will have begun to accept you as perhaps too cautious and unadventurous. Start turning this image that others have of you around by you starting the conversations and the invitations.

Taking risks

Begin by creating mini challenges for yourself on a daily basis. Initially this could be walking the last mile to work, staying on later at work, getting into communication with someone that you have recently had a row with, venturing out more perhaps at weekends – especially to visit friends or family members that you have recently been avoiding.

Focusing

It may sound a boring and tedious exercise but a good old-fashioned 'to do' list is an excellent yangizing exercise. Jot down all the things that you need to complete at home and at work. Make a list of letters you need to write and conversations that you need to complete with others. It is important that you initiate these conversations and do not wait in the yin mode for the telephone to ring.

Sleep

When our condition becomes too yin, it is not uncommon to feel more awake and more inspired around the midnight hour. Unfortunately, this will continue to drain your condition and make you even more yin. Make the effort to be in bed before midnight and up shortly before dawn. For an additional challenge, put aside your alarm clock for ten days while you cultivate an internal discipline for waking naturally and on time.

Avoid long hot baths

These have a profound yinizing effect on your Chi. Definitely avoid a long hot bath immediately after getting up in the morning. The logic is quite simple - you have just emerged from an eight-your yin activity – sleep – only to immerse yourself in a long, hot bath. It will only make you more tired and more yin in this state of Chi. Far better to have a short, warm shower and, if you have the courage, give yourself a blast of cold water at the end!

Chanting and meditation

I have always found that these two exercises have a profoundly yangizing effect upon my Chi. They are simple to practise yet challenging when we feel particularly yin. Often when our condition is too yin we do not feel attracted to the discipline and stillness that these to exercises require.

For both of these exercises you need to sit correctly so that your spine is erect. I particularly recommend the Japanese seated position known as seiza. This is the way that most Japanese sit traditionally at home and you may have seen them take this posture in a Japanese restaurant. Begin by removing your shoes and ensure that your lower body is not too restrained by a tight skirt or tight trousers. Find a suitably soft mat that you can place on the carpet. Slowly bend your knees, coming down so you are kneeling on the mat with your knees and shin bones on the floor and your buttocks sitting on your heels. Have your knees approximately one-fist width apart and make sure that both big toes are resting one upon the other. Stretch your arms high above your head and raise your gaze towards the ceiling. Look directly forward and slowly lower your arms so that your hands rest in your lap. Both palms should be facing upwards. Place the hand that you normally write with underneath your more inactive hand. With your hands cupped in this position in your lap let your thumbs touch. You are now ready to practise either of the two meditations below.

Chanting DO

Sit peacefully in seiza posture for 3 or 4 minutes. Narrow down your eyes so they are almost closed and look at a point on the carpet ahead of you approximately 1 metre/yard away. Breathe gently from your belly, inhaling for 2 seconds, holding the breath for 3 or 4 seconds and then slowly releasing the breath through your mouth for up to 6-8 seconds. Maintain this breathing for 1 or 2 minutes and then on the next out breath chant DO (pronounced Dough). Breathe in as outlined above and as you breathe out continue to chant DO. Repeat this 10-15 times. Notice how the sound seems to emanate from your belly and that after the chanting this area becomes far more warm. You are welcome to chant for longer as this will leave you feeling even more 'grounded' and yang.

Za-Zen meditation

This is a very yangizing form of meditation that requires you to sit in seiza posture and to follow the breathing technique described above. Position yourself 1-2 metres/yards from a blank wall. There is no chanting involved in this meditation, simply sit absolutely still in a relaxed state, gazing at the wall. Any tension that you feel during the exercise you can release with your out breath. Do not allow yourself to linger on any particular thoughts – just be in the present. Initially you can practise this meditation for 5-10 minutes and slowly build it up to 15-20 minutes daily. It is ideally practised shortly after rising and after you have washed but before you eat. Za-Zen has a profoundly yangizing effect as it brings you into the moment. In Japan, if you practise this meditation in a dojo (temple) you may have the extra discipline of the sensei (master) quietly pacing up and down behind a row of students looking for any sign of lapse of concentration. Sensei is looking for any stooping of the shoulders, shaking of the head or glazing over of the eyes. In a traditional dojo he would have a large stick in one hand with which he would either gently tap on your shoulder to remind you to return to the present or yangize you with a swift, sharp strike!

CHI/SPIRIT – TOO YANG

When your chi is highly overcharged, you feel capable of anything and completely unstoppable. In this frame of mind you believe you can take on the world. Everyone else appears too slow, too cautious and wimpish. Imagine being in this state of hyperactivity and being told to relax? When my Chi has become too yang and I am advised to slow down, I inevitably look at my source of advice with a kind of disdain! What's wrong with them, can't they keep up the pace, they need yangizing! If, however, you have come to the conclusion that your way of being – your Chi – has become too yang then try on some of these methods to develop a more yin nature.

Developing your sensitivity

Make the effort to do something everyday that reveals to others the softer, more yin side of your nature. This could involve dressing more casually. You could buy someone a bunch of flowers. You could be more generous with your time to someone near you. Take time out to listen to someone every day. Commit yourself to an act of generosity.

I remembering counselling a gentleman some years ago who was an aggressive property dealer in London. He had a physical problem that was essentially caused by too much yang. One of the general pieces of advice that I gave him was to take up some form of relaxation and to make more effort to be generous in order to resolve his excessively yang qualities. Towards the end of our meeting his mobile telephone rang. He had a quick, fairly abrupt conversation with someone which ended with him saying, 'That's ok, that's ok, that's ok.' He then declared that he had just taken my advice. A prospective buyer had been hassling him all day about the price of a property that he was selling, and he showed that he had just taken my advice by 'giving in' to this man's last offer. I asked him how he felt? Different, he said, and then a large broad grin appeared on his face and for the first time in our conversation he looked completely relaxed.

Be around the yinnie

When we are too yang we inevitably have no time or patience for people who procrastinate and dither. However, they can provide us with the best training in becoming more yin! Think of the most annoyingly yin person that comes to mind, give them a call and arrange to spend some time with them. It could be on a project related to work; the person could be a dithering member of your family or a neighbour who has asked for some help at home, and you have avoided doing this because you know it will mean hours of delay and procrastination. Don't bring your yang to the party, simply be with their way of going about things however frustrating. At the end of the ordeal, what did you learn? If you genuinely listen, observe and get into what they are doing on their level – you will certainly learn a lot about yin.

Shopping

The weekly grocery run is, for my money, one of the most yang-izing experiences on earth! It is not a lot of fun, it is certainly not relaxing, it is a chore. The kind of shopping on which you need to embark is at a purely sensory level. This, for a yang person, is an immense challenge. Drifting aimlessly through your local mall, window shopping, browsing, trying things on, stopping for a cake, cup of tea or a beer, has a very yinizing effect. If you want it to have the maximum effect on you, take with you a guide who absolutely loves this kind of shopping! Don't let your yang get in the way, go with their Chi and their spirit. Stick with it and you have every chance of becoming more yin; fight it and your yang nature will only become more compounded.

Play with a child

The world of a young child, their fantasies, their dreams, their expressions, their imagination and their appetite are all excellent sources of yin. The secret lies in getting in on their level, listening to them. What do they want to do this afternoon? Where would they like to go? What would be their idea of fun? It is not about you going in there as a benevolent aunt or uncle with your idea of what could be fun for them. Let them dictate the pace, let them decide where and what you want to do. Have no agenda of your own, simply be with them and their Chi.

Shiatsu massage

Find a local practitioner who is recommended by a friend and who you can visit two or three times during this ten-day programme. Shiatsu is the Japanese form of massage that is embedded in understanding the body purely in terms of Chi. A good practitioner, during the 1-hour session, has the potential to release all kinds of tension that has built up within your nervous system, muscles and Chi. Their years of exercise can detect where the Chi is too yang and there are many techniques to release that effectively.

Abandon your watch

Time is the yang factor relative to space. Being under constant pressure to meet deadlines, to be at a certain place at a certain time, to have restrictions put upon the length of meetings and conversations, are all intensely yang. When we are over yang we can have a very acute sense of time, knowing for example exactly what time it is and how much time we need to get the job done. People whose Chi is far more yin than yours have a whole different concept of the passing hours. They are generally slower and time moves more slowly for them. Frustrating for a yang person! For the ten-day period my advice is to leave your watch at home. Cover up clocks in your office and put a yellow Post-it note over any digital clocks in your space. Why do you think holidays are so relaxing and yinizing without any constraints of time, commitments for meetings and deadlines to meet?

Sleep

When we are very wired up and our Chi is too yang we often need very little sleep. Continually having very little sleep, working hard and impatiently inevitably makes us feel that it is normal to sleep only a few hours a night. Anyone who sleeps any more than us is definitely too yin! Try and have a hot, relaxing bath before bed – if it is going to be a long bath put some sea salt in so that you do not leech away too many vital minerals. If, despite this advice, you still wake up very early, then rather than going back to sleep or getting up to write a business report at 6 a.m. use this time creatively in a more yin fashion. Yinizing and relaxing activities include making love, a long gentle walk, writing a poem or a diary, creating something artistic or listening to relaxing music.

DIET

'It is by means of food that man's body is sustained, and it is by means of food that the quality and direction of life are determined. Preparing the food that sustains "tomorrow's life" is a creative act; to be successful in this art one needs deep understanding, subtle delicacy and true dedication.'

Lima Ohsawa

Cooking intuitively

I began to study macrobiotic cookery in 1976 and found the changes in my vitality, stamina and outlook changed dramatically within several weeks. Macrobiotics is essentially applying the yin/yang principle to what you eat, how you prepare it and how you adjust what you eat to suit your current condition. With time and practice it becomes second nature. The ideas presented in this section on diet are based on the principles of macrobiotics with a broader perspective on cooking styles and ingredients which will allow transition to these ideas without too violent a swing from what you were used to previously.

Just as important as 'what' you eat is 'how' you cook. For me, cooking is a form of meditation. Minimize any distractions while you are preparing the food and take a moment to assess what your needs are and what you want to prepare before you set out. If you are straight in from work, take a shower or relax before you start to create a meal. The real discipline of cooking is the capacity to be totally calm and totally occupied on what you are doing for the 15-45-minute period in which you prepare a meal. Even with a busy lifestyle it is worth putting aside time every day to prepare at least one meal. With careful planning and foresight, some elements can be put aside for tomorrow's lunch box or used as the basis for a soup next day.

Chewing

Many of the ingredients here are simple, old-fashioned, peasant foods. As with all traditional foods we need to chew them very well. These foods are not pre-digested as with so many refined products that are available today. Chewing can bring us into a more relaxed state; we are able to appreciate more the subtleties of taste and texture, and it is a chance in our busy lives to take a moment to relax and reflect. Over the years, I have noticed that people that chew slowly and chew well seem more calm and unhurried whereas individuals who gulp their food are far more hyperactive.

The principles

As I explained in Chapter 3, the knowledge and use of certain principles and utilizing them in the preparation of our food can transform any ingredient to suit our current condition.

Fire

The higher and the more active the flame, the more yang the result. A low flame creates a more yin effect, no flame (raw food) is the ultimate expression of a yin cooking preparation.

Time

The longer you cook your food the more yang it becomes (roasting, baking). The shorter the cooking the more yin the preparation style (steaming, blanching).

Pressure

The more pressure we bring into our cooking the more yang the result. Examples include the use of a pressure cooker, heavy casserole pots with the lid on, baking and pickling. Little or no pressure is when we cook without a lid and use the burners rather than the oven.

Salt

Salt is a very yang ingredient that human beings have sought and used for thousands of years. Salt as a mineral is fundamental to our electrolyte balance – too much or too little can cause problems.

The more salt we use in our cooking the more yang the result.

The less salt or abstinence from salt creates a more yin style of cooking.

In all the ideas and recipes here sea salt is recommended, but only in cooking. I never recommend it raw at the table.

The ingredients

Quality

To maximize the positive effect of what you eat on your blood during this programme, go for the best quality of food that you can find. Ideally, this needs to be wholesome, natural foods, preferably organic; all fruits, vegetables, salads and fish need to be as fresh as possible.

Variety

Truly this quality is the spice of life. Eating the same old foods day in, day out will inevitably lead to a lack of spark in your energy. Make sure that you integrate a variety of colours, tastes, textures, flavours and cooking styles.

Foods to reduce

Some foods require a lot more effort to digest than others. For the purpose of this ten-day programme I am suggesting that you leave out certain foods which are either harder to digest or have potential to change your Chi too quickly or too violently. This is not to say that these foods are 'wrong' but that if you wish to benefit from the concept that you can create a quiet space within yourself over this time then it is better to avoid the following:

Raw salt (that is, salt not used in cooking), eggs, all animal food and animal fats, all dairy products, sugar, coffee, refined carbohydrate (white bread, pastry, etc) and any food product or beverage that contains sugar.

Once you have decided whether your condition is more yin or more yang there are two choices you could make regarding making a shift in your diet. The first is to bring as many 'yang' qualities as you can to your cooking styles and ingredients – or vice versa for a yang condition. Even minor changes will help.

The second approach is to adopt the recipes that I have selected from a macrobiotic perspective and used myself over the past twenty years. If you find the ingredients unfamiliar and you are very pressed for time, this second approach may be challenging even though the benefits are more rewarding. The choice is yours!

Here are some qualities if you wish to make a shift toward yin or yang without using unfamiliar ingredients:

ADDING MORE YANG

- More cooking (fire)
- More savoury dishes
- More warm/hot foods
- Hot breakfast rather than cold
  – porridge/toast/kipper
- Hot soup with lunch
- Stir-fried meals
- Well-cooked stews
- Hot evening meal
- Warm/hot desserts
- Hot beverages

ADDING MORE YIN

- Less cooking (leaning towards raw/blanching)
- Sweeter/spicy dishes
- Cooler/cold dishes
- Light/cool breakfasts

- fruit/cereals/sweet porridge/muesli
- Lighter lunch
  - salads
  - pasta
  - very little or no animal protein
- Lightly cooked evening meal
  - cool/cold desserts
- Beverages that are either cool or cooling (Herb Teas)

YIN APPROACHES TO COOKING – WHEN YOU'RE TOO YANG

Breakfast

SWEET PORRIDGE (serves 2)

1 cup/100g/3½oz porridge oat flakes (not the pre-cooked sort)
3-4 cups*/about 840ml/1⅓ pints spring water
small handful of washed raisins
pinch sea salt
malt extract
soya milk

Place all the ingredients in the heaviest pot that you have. Bring the oats to the boil, turn down the flame and constantly stir for 3 minutes. Let it summer for 7-10 minutes, stirring from time to time.

Eat this while it is still hot, adding malt extract as a sweetener and 1-2 tablespoons/15-30ml soya milk.

*For convenience any cup may be used provided it contains 210-235ml/7-8fl oz. However, please be sure to use the same cup for all ingredients in that recipe, and do not mix cup and other weighed measures.

WHOLEMEAL TOAST

Lightly toast 2 slices of the best quality wholemeal bread that you can buy. Spread over a little tahini or smooth peanut butter or a good quality soya-based spread. To add sweetness you can use any sugar-free jam or marmalade.

MUESLI

Choose a good quality muesli base in which preferably any grain flakes are toasted. Pre-soak the muesli in apple juice, spring water or soya milk. Add half a cup/about 3½oz/100g of fresh seasonal local fruit that is diced or sliced.

HERBAL TEAS

Camomile tea – relaxing
Mint tea – refreshing

Midday meal

CAULIFLOWER SOUP (SERVES 4)

1 small cauliflower
4 cups/840ml/1⅓ pints spring water
½ tsp sea salt
2 whole spring onions, chopped
½ cup/100g/3½oz carrot, finely sliced
¼ lemon
garnish – parsley

Wash all the vegetables very well and chop the cauliflower into small pieces. Combine the water, sea salt and cauliflower in a pot and bring to the boil. Allow it to simmer gently until the cauliflower is soft. At this point add the spring onions together with the carrot. Simmer for another 2 minutes. Finally, before turning off the soup add the juice of the ¼ lemon. Garnish with three sprigs of parsley.

BONITO BROTH (serves 4)

4 cups/840ml/1⅓ pints spring water
pinch sea salt
4-inch/10cm strip of kombu (dried sea vegetable)
3 tbsp/45ml of bonito flakes
½ cup/100g/3½oz sliced onions
2 whole spring onions
1 tbsp/15ml shoyu
garnish – slice of lemon or sprig parsley, chopped chives,
    sprinkling of spring onion

Put the water, sea salt and the washed strip of kombu together with the bonito flakes in a suitable pot. Bring this to the boil. At this point add the onions and wait until they have turned translucent (2-3 minutes). Now add the 2 spring onions chopped into thirds, together with the shoyu as seasoning. Simmer for a further 2 minutes. Sieve this stock and garnish the broth with a half moon slice of lemon, a sprig of parsley, chopped chives or chopped spring onions.

RICE SALAD (serves 2)

2 cups/440ml/16 fl oz cold cooked short-grain brown rice,
    about 1 cup/200g/7oz raw (see p. 211)
1 spring onion
1 small cucumber pickle (gherkin)
½ cup/100g/3½oz diced raw carrot
½ cup/100g/3½oz blanched broccoli
3 tbsp/30ml roasted sunflower seeds
parsley
1 tsp shoyu
1 tsp brown rice vinegar

Place the cool brown rice in a large enough bowl and mix in the diced carrot, a finely chopped spring onion, a diced pickled cucumber, the blanched cold broccoli, the sunflower seeds, the finely chopped parsley and shoyu and rice vinegar to taste. Mix it well.

BLANCHED VEGETABLE SALAD (serves 2)

½ cup/100g/3½oz Chinese cabbage
½ cup/100g/3½oz sliced carrot
½ cup/100g/3½oz chopped celery
½ bunch washed fresh watercress

Bring 2-3 inches/5-7ml water to the boil with a small pinch of sea salt. Keep the flames as high as possible. Drop in the vegetables and wait for the water to come back to a vigorous boil. After 2 minutes (no longer) pour the contents through a sieve, keeping the vegetable stock and then immediately rinsing the vegetables under flowing cold water. You can add the water from the vegetables to a soup stock and you could dress this salad with a few drops of brown rice vinegar or shoyu.

UDON NOODLES WITH TOFU AND BONITO BROTH (serves 4)

1 packet/250g/8½oz udon noodles
1 cup/200g/7oz fresh tofu cut in quarter-inch/½cm cubes
4 cups/840ml/1⅓ pints bonito broth

Cook the udon noodles with a pinch of sea salt following the supplier's instructions. Bring the bonito broth to the boil and add the cubed tofu. When the tofu begins to rise to the surface it will be ready. Sieve the udon noodles and rinse them briefly under cold running water. Place in a bowl and pour the broth and tofu over the noodles, garnishing with either parsley, chives, spring onions or half a slice of lemon.

UDON NOODLE SALAD

1 packet/250g/8½oz udon noodles
½ cup/100g/3½oz diced, blanched carrots
1 spring onion, chopped
½ cup/100g/3½oz chopped celery
handful of washed raisins
handful of roasted sunflower seeds
parsley
shoyu
rice vinegar

Cook the udon noodles with a pinch of sea salt according to the manufacturer's instructions. When they are ready rinse them in a sieve under cold running water. Mix in the diced vegetables, the finely chopped parsley, spring onion, raisins, sunflower seeds and complete by adding shoyu and rice vinegar to taste.

GLAZED PEARS (serves 2)

2 fresh hard pears
½ cup/100ml/3½fl oz fresh apple juice
pinch sea salt
½ tsp Kuzu or ¼ tsp arrowroot
garnish – chopped roasted hazelnuts or walnuts

Cut the pears into quarters and remove their cores. Boil them in a mixture of the apple juice and 1 cup/210ml/7fl oz of spring water and a few grains of sea salt. Cook them until they are almost soft. Mix either the kuzu or the arrowroot into 3 tbsp/45ml cold water. Drain off most of the cooking juice until approximately ½ cup/100ml/3½oz is left. Add the thickening agent and stir over the heat for a further 3-4 minutes. Place the pears and the glazing in bowls and garnish with the chopped nuts.

CEREAL GRAIN COFFEE

There are many different brands available. They can be made from barley, chicory or dandelion.

Evening meal

MISO SOUP (serves 4)

4 cups/840ml/1⅓ pints spring water
7cm/3 inches dried wakame seaweed
½ cup/100g/3½oz onion, finely sliced
½ cup/100g/3½oz carrot, sliced
2 to 4 tsp/10-20fl oz miso
1 spring onion, finely sliced
½ cup/100g/3½oz fresh tofu, cut into ¼ inch/½cm cubes
   (optional)
garnish – 1 spring onion

Begin by bringing the water to the boil. While you are waiting for this to happen soak the wakame for 5 minutes until it opens up. When the water begins to boil add the onions followed by the wakame having first removed the 'spine' and chopped it into 2cm/1in strips. When this combination is boiling add the carrots for a further 4 mins. Remove ½ cup/100ml/3½fl oz of the broth and add to it between ½-1tsp of miso for each remaining cup/200ml/7fl oz of broth. Dissolve the miso into the ½ cup of stock and replace it in the soup. Let this gently simmer for a further 2 mins.

If you are using the tofu, add it when you put in the carrots.

Garnish with finely chopped spring onion.

This miso soup is ideally taken daily and will keep in the fridge for 2-3 days. Do not reheat the whole pot each time, just remove enough for each meal, and do not take more than one helping each day.

BROWN RICE (serves 4)

3 cups/550g/1¼lbs washed organic short-grain brown rice
4 cups/840ml/1⅓ pints spring water
pinch sea salt
flame deflector

Wash the brown rice extremely well and place in a heavy pot
with the spring water and no more than ½ tsp sea salt. Make sure
that you have a good tight-fitting lid for this pot. Bring the rice
to a boil on a fairly high flame. At this point turn the flame down
and place a metal flame deflector between the flame and the base
of the pot. Cook very slowly for 45-50 minutes and resist the
temptation to stir!

Turn off the flame and leave for 10 mins before removing the
pot and serving the rice.

Brown rice will keep for at least 3 days. It will dry out if you
place it in a refrigerator. The best solution is to place it in a
mildly oiled wooden fruit bowl, cover it with a clean, slightly
damp cloth and place it in a cool part of your kitchen.

UDON NOODLES

Bring one packet of udon noodles to the boil in spring water and
a pinch of sea salt. Follow the manufacturer's instructions as to
the length of time. Pour them out into a sieve and cool them
under plenty of cold running water. Udon noodles will keep
fresh in the fridge for 2-3 days.

ADUKI BEAN CASSEROLE (serves 4)

1 cup/200g/7oz aduki beans
12cm/5-inch piece of dried kombu
sea salt
3 cups (about 300g/11oz) diced carrot, parsnips or pumpkin (or
    a mixture of these)
spring water

Wash the aduki beans and kombu well. Soak the beans and kombu in the spring water for 2-3 hours. Chop the kombu into 2cm/1-inch squares.

Place the kombu at the bottom of the pot together with the chopped vegetables, adding the beans on top. Add water (including the soaking water) until this mixture is covered by approximately 1cm/½in. Cook the casserole until the beans are soft (40-60 minutes). For the last 10 mins of cooking season with a light sprinkling of sea salt.

It is important that the beans are properly cooked. A good test is if you can place one of the beans on the tip of your tongue and crush it fairly easily against the roof of your mouth. If they are hard and chewy, they need further cooking. This stew will keep for at least 2 days in the refrigerator. The more you reheat it or the longer you cook it the more delicious it becomes. You can also use this stew as the basis for a soup the next day.

WHITE FISH (serves 4)

170-220g/6-8oz cod, haddock, sole or plaice
sesame oil
shoyu

Wash the fish well, dry it with a cloth and then rub in a mixture of sesame oil and shoyu. Grill the fish until it is cooked.

Garnish with lemon or parsley or add a few drops of ginger juice extracted from peeled, fresh raw-root ginger.

STEAMED GREENS

2 cups/225g/8oz sliced or chopped green vegetables (kale or watercress, Chinese cabbage or spring greens)

You need a pot with a tight-fitting lid. If you do not have a vegetable steamer, simply bring 1cm/½ inch mildly salted water to a vigorous boil. Put in the vegetables, replace the tight-fitting lid and leave for 2-5 mins depending on the texture of the vegetables. A stainless steel vegetable steamer is beneficial. The same general principles apply.

Serve these hot with your noodle or brown rice dish and your protein dish of fish or aduki beans.

SAUTÉ VEGETABLES (serves 2)

sesame oil
½ cup/100g/3½oz finely cut carrot
½ cup/100g/3½oz finely cut onion
¾ cup/100g/3½oz cabbage or Chinese cabbage

Brush a heavy pan with sesame oil. Put the pan on a low flame and begin by sautéing the onions until they become transparent. At this stage add a few drops of shoyu or a small pinch of sea salt. Add the other vegetables and 1-2 tbsp/15-30ml water. Simmer for 4-8 mins.

The vegetables should be crispy, colourful and cooked.

AMASAKE WITH GINGER (serves 4)

Amasake is a delicious, creamy rice-based dessert. It is made from the fermentation process that is one of the steps in the production of the Japanese wine saki and is available in many health food shops. Place 1 cup/210ml/7fl oz of amasake in a suitable pot with ½ cup/110ml/3½fl oz spring water. Peel a small piece of fresh raw-root ginger, grate it finely and squeeze out ¼ tsp juice. Add this juice to the water and amasake and slowly heat the mixture stirring it constantly. Only let it simmer for 1 or 2 mins and enjoy this while it is hot.

Eating out – yin ideas

It is not always convenient to cook for yourself 3 times a day and it is possible to 'forage' for a snack or a meal from the variety in our city centres. The secret lies in finding the best quality available. Is it clean, is it fresh, do the chefs look bright, happy and energetic? Have you had a good recommendation from a friend? Here are some ideas that you could utilize. Don't forget that the best food is always cooked with your own love, patience and focus.

STUFFED PITTA BREAD

See if you can find wholemeal pitta bread and have it filled with fresh salad and freshly made hummus.

SANDWICH BARS

Take-away restaurants can often provide you with a bean salad, a green salad or a fresh fruit salad.

JAPANESE FOODS

A quick and refreshing meal can often be found at the sushi bar. Always insist on the best quality. Try sushi, white rice wrapped in nori seaweed with a filling of either pickle or cucumber. Ask for ohshitshi – cold, blanched green vegetables.

For a really refreshing snack try zaru soba. This dish is made from buckwheat noodles that have been cooked and allowed to drain and cool. They are served cold, sometimes even on a bed of ice, with a deliciously refreshing and tangy dipping sauce made from primarily shoyu, spring onions and a unique form of horseradish known as washabi. This is a very good pick-me-up.

YANG APPROACHES TO COOKING – WHEN YOU'RE TOO YIN

Breakfast

PORRIDGE (serves 2)

1 cup/100g/3½oz porridge oat flakes (not the pre-cooked sort)
3-4 cups/about 840ml/1⅓ pints spring water
pinch sea salt
garnish – gomashio*

Place the contents into a heavy pan and slowly bring to the boil, stirring from time to time. When the porridge is boiling turn the flame down, place on a flame deflector and gently cook for a further 10-15 mins stirring every 3 or 4 mins. Sprinkle up to a tsp/5ml of gomashio.

*Gomashio is a delicious condiment made by roasting one part of sea salt with 20 parts of washed sesame seeds. Lightly roast these in a heavy pan until the sesame seeds turn a golden brown and give off a nutty aroma. When the mixture is cool enough, lightly grind them together until 80 per cent of the seeds are crushed. You can store this mixture in an airtight jar to add to your porridge or any dish that contains either noodles or grain.

SCRAMBLED TOFU (serves 1)

sunflower or sesame oil
110-160g/4-6 oz fresh tofu
½ cup/100g/3½oz diced onion
3 small mushrooms, chopped
shoyu

Take a heavy pan and lightly brush the inside with oil. Begin by sautéing the onions and mushrooms adding a few drops of shoyu to bring out the liquid. When they are soft add the tofu, crumbling it with a wooden spoon as you stir. Add 3 tbsp/50ml water and cook on a low flame preferably with the lid on for at least 8 mins.

Ideally, you need to 'cook off' all the excess water. For the final few minutes of cooking remove the lid and season with shoyu. Serve this hot on fresh, lightly toasted wholemeal bread.

KIPPER

A good fishmonger will be able to provide you with naturally smoked kippers. You can either grill these slowly under a low flame or place them in a stainless steel vegetable steamer and steam them with a tight-fitting lid for at least 8 mins. Garnish with parsley and serve them with a small wedge of lemon.

MISO SOUP

Miso soup, or indeed any soup, for breakfast would not be the natural choice for most Westerners. However, it is not uncommon elsewhere in the world for people to enjoy a hot, savoury breakfast to start the day. In many cultures this includes soups, stews and different forms of grain-based gruel. The heat and the savoury quality of this kind of breakfast has the potential to bring you into focus very quickly.

See recipe on p. 210 – you can include the diced, cooked tofu if you wish.

CEREAL GRAIN COFFEE

There are a variety of beverages based on barley, chicory or dandelion. Try a few from your local health food shop

Midday meal

CREAMY CARROT SOUP (serves 4)

4 medium-sized carrots, cut into large chunks
5 cups/1¼l/2 pints spring water
¼ cup/25g/1oz oat flakes
pinch sea salt
miso
12cm/5-inch strip of kombu
parsley for garnish

Wash the kombu and place it with the carrots in the spring water
with a pinch of sea salt. Bring to the boil, cover with a lid and
leave to simmer for 35 mins. Slowly stir in the oat flakes and
continue to stir until they become creamy. Allow to simmer
gently for a further 15 mins adding ½-1 tbsp/8-15ml miso to
taste. Remember to dilute the miso in ½ cup of soup stock before
you add it to the pan.
    Garnish with parsley.

BEAN SOUP (serves 4)

1 cup/200g/7oz dried beans (green or brown lentils, aduki
    beans, chick peas, black beans, red kidney beans or a
    mixture)
2 sliced onions
pinch sea salt
2 finely diced carrots
shoyu
parsley

Wash the beans and allow them to soak for 2-3 hours. Lentils
often need less time than this. Sauté the onions and carrots in a
small amount of sesame or sunflower oil. When they are soft add
4 cups/840ml/1⅓ pints spring water and the beans. Bring the

soup to a boil, removing any froth that may appear. Turn down the flame and let the soup simmer for at least 40 mins. In the last 3 mins season with a small amount of shoyu. Garnish with finely chopped parsley.

DEEP-FRIED RICE BALLS (serves 2)

2 cups/440ml/16fl oz cool left-over brown rice, about 1 cup/200g/7oz raw (see p. 211)
½ cup/100g/3½oz finely diced blanched carrots
1 tbsp/15ml finely chopped chives
½ cup/100g/3½oz finely cut sautéed onion
wholemeal flour, breadcrumbs or sesame seeds
shoyu

Place the first four ingredients in a fairly large mixing bowl and work them together with your clean hands. Add a few drops of shoyu. Dampen your hands under a running tap and take a handful of the rice mixture. Squeeze it into a ball that can fit neatly inside the palms of your hands. Dust the surface with either wholemeal flour, breadcrumbs or crushed, roasted sesame seeds. Heat almost 7cm/3 inches sesame oil in a heavy pan. Keep a close eye on it. To check when the oil is ready for deep frying, throw in one grain of cooked rice. If it bounces up to the surface quickly and sizzles, the oil are ready. Gently place in the rice balls and cook them until they are golden brown. Allow them to drain and eat them while they are hot with a few drops of shoyu.

These can also be eaten cold.

STIR-FRIED RICE OR STIR-FRIED NOODLES (serves 4)

1 pkt/250g/8½oz soba noodles or udon noodles, cooked and cooled
or

2 cups/440ml/16fl oz cooked cold brown rice, about
   1 cup/200g/7oz raw (see p. 211)
½ cup/100g/3½oz sliced onions
½ cup/100g/4oz finely chopped carrot
1 bunch chopped watercress
sesame oil
shoyu
tofu, fish or prawns
garnish – 2 finely chopped spring onions

Find a frying pan or preferably a wok. Lightly brush the surface
with sesame oil. When the oil is hot add the onions and a few
drops of shoyu. When the onions become translucent add the
carrots and whichever protein you wish to use (tofu, fish or
prawns). Keep the flame high and keep stirring vigorously. You
may find you need to add a few tbsp water. As the vegetables
become softer add either the rice or the noodles. Keep stirring
vigorously until the protein source is cooked. For the final 2
mins add the chopped watercress and a few more drops of shoyu.
   Serve hot and garnish with the spring onions.

VEGETABLES

It is best to avoid eating left-over vegetables. They lose their
freshness, vitality and Chi very quickly. If you are having a
simple lunch of soup and bread or you only have time for a rice
ball, make sure that you do include a portion of vegetables. It
could be a blanched vegetable dish (page 208), a small salad or
some steamed greens.

RICE PUDDING (serves 4)

2 cups/440ml/16fl oz cooked left-over brown rice, about 1
   cup/200g/7oz raw (see p. 211)
a handful of washed raisins
2 tbsp/30ml tahini

½ cup/100ml/3½fl oz soya milk
3 tbsp/45ml barley malt

Begin by placing the cooked rice and a small amount of spring water in a heavy pot. Bring this to the boil, slowly turn down the flame and add the raisins, barley malt, tahini and soya milk. Stir it well. Allow this to simmer until the fluid has been absorbed and the rice is creamy.

Alternatively, when you have brought the ingredients to the boil you can place the casserole pot in the oven and bake for at least 45 mins.

This rice pudding will keep for 2 days in the fridge provided it was made originally with freshly cooked rice.

KUKICHA

Sometimes known as bancha twig tea, kukicha is a simple tea made from the twigs of the kukicha plant. It has a very mild taste and has little or no traces of caffeine or tannin. You can buy it in a health food shop, usually in twig form. However, it is not possible to purchase kukicha in a tea bag variation. Kukicha can be boiled again and again and again and is still refreshing.

Bring 6 cups/1¼l/2½ pints spring water to the boil and sprinkle approximately 2 tbsp/30ml of kukicha twigs on the surface. Simmer this for 5-10 mins, simply strain out a cup of the tea and drink it hot, warm or even cold. You can reheat this many times, even adding a little more water each time.

Evening meal

MISO SOUP

(See p. 210.)

SAVOURY SNACK ON TOAST

Try one of the following ideas on lightly toasted good quality wholemeal toast:
smoked salmon
tuna fish pâté
vegetable or mushroom pâté from a health food shop
grilled sardines

PAELLA

225g/8oz prawns, cooked
110g/4oz shrimps, cooked
450g/1 lb mussels or clams
1½ cups/275g/10oz basmati rice
sesame oil
1 clove garlic
2 onions, finely chopped
1 red pepper, finely chopped
juice from ½ lemon
saffron
parsley

Wash all the seafood very well. Peel half of the prawns and boil the peelings for 20 mins in mildly salty water. Add the mussels and simmer until the shells open. Strain the stock through a fine sieve to use for cooking the rice later. Set the mussels aside.

Find a wide, shallow heavy cast-iron pot with a lid. Oil it well with sesame oil. Sauté the onions, the garlic and chopped red pepper. When the vegetables are soft add 4½ cups/1¾ pints fish stock and the rice. Bring to the boil and gently simmer for 20 mins. After 20 mins add the shelled prawns, shrimps, shelled mussels, clams, or any other sea food. Add a little saffron and lemon juice and continue to cook for 3-4 mins. Serve garnished with plenty of fresh parsley and any remaining unpeeled prawns. Choose one of the vegetable dishes from p. 208 or p. 212 to complement the meal.

MILLET MASH (serves 4)

2 cups/420g/14oz millet
pinch sea salt
1 cauliflower

Wash and strain the millet. Place it in a heavy cast-iron pot or frying pan and gently roast it, constantly stirring it with a wooden spatula. Wait until it has gone a golden brown colour. Add the roasted millet to 3 cups/630ml/1¼ pints water and a pinch of sea salt. Bring to the boil and allow to simmer gently for 20 mins. Meanwhile clean and prepare one small cauliflower. Chop it into small pieces and drop it into a generous amount of water with a pinch of sea salt. When the cauliflower is soft, add it to the millet (you may need a little of the cauliflower's cooking water as well) and mash them together with a potato masher. Serve hot with mushroom gravy.

MUSHROOM GRAVY (serves 2)

6 small fresh mushrooms, finely chopped
¼ cup/50g/2oz unbleached wheat flour
sea salt
sesame oil
shoyu
vegetable stock
kuzu or arrowroot

Use a heavy pot to make this gravy. Begin by gently heating ½ tbsp/8ml sesame oil. Add the flour and stir it well for at least 6–7 mins. When it turns a golden colour and smells cooked, remove it from the heat and allow it to cool down.

In another pan, sauté the mushrooms in sesame oil, adding a few grains of sea salt to bring out the liquid in the mushrooms. When they are almost soft add the flour to the pan with the mushrooms together with 3 cups/630ml/1¼ pints vegetable stock. (This could be the liquid left over from steamed greens or boiled or blanched vegetables.) Stir the gravy vigorously and when smooth add ½ tsp kuzu or ¼ tsp arrowroot (diluted in 3 tbsp/45ml cold liquid). Simmer for 3-4 mins and season further with sea salt or shoyu if necessary.

Serve this on the millet mash or use it with the deep fried rice balls mentioned on p. 218.

MILLET CROQUETTES

left-over millet mash
wholemeal flour, breadcrumbs or sesame seeds
sesame oil

Millet is a delicious grain and lends itself well to deep frying. With your hands wet form small balls or croquettes with the millet. Dust them in either breadcrumbs, flour or roasted, crushed sesame seeds.

Bring the sesame oil to a high temperature, dropping a small piece of cooked millet into the oil and noticing when it returns rapidly to the surface. When this occurs you are ready to begin deep frying. Cook for 3-4 mins and serve hot.

These croquettes are delicious with any of the vegetable dishes mentioned on pp. 208 or 212.

PANCAKES (serves 4)

approx ½ litre/scant pint spring water (half of which can be
    sparkling)
2 cups/350g/12oz unbleached flour
1 tsp/5ml kuzu or ½ tsp arrowroot
zest of ½ a lemon
sesame oil
pinch sea salt

Put approximately 1 tbsp sesame oil at the bottom of your

mixing bowl. Add flour, lemon zest and pinch sea salt. Dissolve the kuzu or arrowroot in 2 tbsp/30ml cold water. Add this to the flour. Gently pour in the spring water, adding enough to create a thick creamy consistency, then whisk and stir vigorously until you have a smooth batter. Leave to rest in the fridge for half an hour.

Find a suitable heavy pan and generously oil the surface with sesame oil. Have a fairly high flame and when the oil is smoking add just enough batter to cover the surface of the pan. When it bubbles and blisters briskly turn it over and cook the other side.

Fill these pancakes with:
   sugar-free jam
   barley malt and lemon juice
   or a good quality sugar-free apple sauce

BAKED APPLES (serves 2)

2 medium sized apples
tahini
miso
raisins

Wash and core 2 medium sized apples. Fill the centre with a mixture of washed raisins with a little miso and tahini. Oil a baking tray and bake at Gas Mark 4/180°C/350°F until they are soft (about 40 mins).

Most wholefood shops can supply you with alternative forms of egg-free and dairy-free custard – for example, soya custard. This can be served either hot or cold. There are also soya-based yoghurt products which will complement this hot dessert.

Eating out

There are times when it is just not possible to cook a meal. Rather than be a 'victim' of your circumstances, be guided by yin/yang principles in deciding what and where to eat. If you look around, there is plenty of choice. Here are some suggestions to help you out.

VEGETABLE SOUP

Almost any restaurant can supply you with a soup of the day – always ask the waiter when it was made.

FISH AND RICE AND VEGETABLES

Many Mediterranean and Middle Eastern restaurants prepare fish and rice and vegetables in a fairly simple manner. You can always request that they do not cover the dish with cheese or butter.

STIR-FRIED RICE OR STIR-FRIED NOODLES

These dishes are fairly widely available but always enquire whether it will be made with monosodium glutamate, then request that the chef leaves out this ingredient. In Chinese restaurants they know it as 'taste'. Ask the chef to prepare your food with no 'taste'!

JAPANESE FOOD

Very warming dishes that you can have include buckwheat noodles (soba noodles) in broth with either deep fried vegetables or deep fried sea food. They can also provide a very warming dish that you can share with others known as nabe. This is where you cook fish and vegetables at your table, to go with any rice or noodles that you have ordered.

VEGETARIAN RESTAURANTS

There is a tendency towards extreme cooking styles in

vegetarian restaurants. The food is either completely raw or very, very well cooked. However, there is invariably a soup of the day and some kind of vegetable bake, casserole or stew. Just try to avoid foods that look like they have been lying there for several hours or have been overcooked (excessive yang).

Conclusion

Apart from the vegetable dishes, the recipes I have given you lend themselves to being either kept in the refrigerator or reheated and used the following day. You can also invent variations around the themes I have mentioned. For example, choose a bigger variety of vegetables than those that I have listed. There are also many more fish, salad ingredients and fruits.

It is not my intention to overburden you with too much time on cooking during the 10-day programme. However, I firmly believe that food has a very profound effect for transformation upon us all. It is after all drawn directly from our environment, and it is from food that we create our blood, nourish our internal organs and refresh our Chi, which is all reflected in how we feel and respond to what is going on around us. If the exercise serves to make you more aware of what you eat and in the long term you begin to take notice of your food and how it is prepared then it has served a valuable purpose.

The less practice you have had in cooking, the more capable you are of taking on a new or different perspective on the art. Try to show an expert how to cook in a totally different way and you will cause confusion. Remember that the key to success with any programme is variety. And please chew well.

9

Where to Go
from Here

Congratulations on completing your version of the 10-day re-balancing programme. At this point it is worth taking time to review how you feel. Think back to the self-assessment check-list that you completed on p. 123 in Chapter 6 and make a note of what improvements you now notice. As with any course of action that involves a change, initially things can look worse before they improve. The frustration, the mistakes, the additional commitments and the unusual variety of tasks to take on board, naturally contribute to feelings of unease. However, after 5 or 6 days, as you got into the rhythm of the programme you will have noticed signs of improvement and change. These changes could be in your physical condition, your ability to deal with pressure, feeling the benefits of enhancing your home environment, noticing how you respond in work and social situations and benefits you observe from paying closer attention to what you eat and how you prepare it.

Remind yourself at this stage also of the visualization exercise in Chapter 7. How did you see yourself in the future? Are you living into this dream at the moment or has it even manifested? Are you still in touch with that dream and is it becoming reality by the day?

What changes will you continue in the future? Perhaps some of the ideas in the programme have inspired you either to find out more or to continue the practice. Try to commit yourself to carrying on at least one of the ideas within the programme. The real freedom to be gained from developing any of these aspects of change beyond the ten-day programme is to discover different perspectives on the idea and constantly try to improve your understanding of the subject.

Congratulate yourself!

It is really worth acknowledging to yourself what you have undertaken. Essentially you decided for yourself whether your current condition was yin or yang, you assessed which area of your life needed working on and it was you who concluded what you needed to do.

Have other people commented that you seem more alert or more relaxed, more flexible, more open? Have guests said your home feels different when they enter? Have work colleagues found you more creative or energetic since you completed the programme? Has your lover found you more attractive? Are colleagues starting to notice that you are on time for meetings or that you are getting the job done without too much fuss? Positive comments from friends, families, lovers and colleagues of a positive nature are all forms of congratulations that you can enjoy.

We are always re-balancing

Yin and yang can provide you with a fascinating and endless model for understanding change. Naturally, the driving force for this principle is that you and I are living in a changing environment and that we ourselves are in a constant state of change. By eliminating extreme yin or extreme yang qualities in our diet, our lifestyle, our activity and our work, we can minimize the swings and shifts that we feel within our own condition. But it would be hopelessly boring to remain completely 'centred' or 'balanced' for the rest of our lives! We need dynamism, we need stimulation and we need to harness change creatively rather than be the victim of it.

Remember that what you designed from this programme, for

this occasion, will not necessarily work next time. Your condition in a month or two will undoubtedly be different. So just because some aspect of the programme worked for you this time it will not necessarily do so on the next occasion. Next time, go through the assessment checklist in Chapter 6 and review it carefully based on how you are feeling then.

The unique feature of this re-balancing programme is that you can return to it time and time again. You may want to assess yourself annually, or at a change of season, at a time when you feel under enormous pressure or when you are considering moving or changing your job. Simplifying your life for these ten days gives you fresh access to your intuition, allowing you to make decisions and judgements that are clear and uncluttered by too many distractions. Essentially, it is the quality of our intuition that dictates the life we create. Getting a handle on 'who you are' and 'where you are' at important turning points in life is essential. Instead of consulting an oracle, a counsellor or an advisor you can simply listen to yourself. Ten days is a realistic and optimum period to regenerate and re-balance your intuition.

Intuition

We all have a tremendous capacity for intuition, but I believe that we do not trust or train this inherent quality. I also believe that intuition has a biological basis. This means that when our health and our lives are more 'balanced' we have a greater capacity to rely on the accuracy of our intuition to form sound judgements and clear navigational perspectives in our life. But if, for example, our condition is too 'yin' – manifesting as feeling tired, withdrawn, protective and unadventurous, then naturally our 'intuition' will be coloured by our condition, and rather than seeking to engage in activities to redress the imbalance, we invariably set out to create the same imbalances. It is rather like having a compass with an error of 10 degrees. We are always going to be 10 degrees off-course!

I believe that regaining your intuition through the steps of this programme can lead to a life that offers you great freedom, health and an appetite for more!

Finding out more

The ideas in this programme are drawn primarily from the wisdom of oriental practices. The programme consists of a number of exercises, recipes, oriental philosophy, Feng Shui and traditional oriental medical principles as well as some Western self-development ideas. If any of these experiences or insights have left you hungry for more, please look at the resource section at the back of the book for further reading and educational support. Any one of the areas can provide you with an Aladdin's cave of ideas and tools for self-discovery. The beauty of all these systems is that essentially they all come from the same stable. Each has an underlying basis of yin and yang, together with a profound appreciation of the importance of Chi/spirit. It is my wish that this book should leave you with a greater appetite for discovery than you had when you first picked it up!

Freedom

The most powerful benefit that we can enjoy from sharpening our intuition is the capacity to enjoy our freedom from previous patterns. This freedom gives us independence and the opportunity to create the life we want. However, real freedom generated by yourself requires some discipline. Discipline in this sense does not imply rigidity, inflexibility and adherence to a set of rules. Discipline is about being in tune and in harmony with ourselves, our surroundings and other people. The discipline involved is simple – live in harmony with the seasons; live in harmony with your family and work colleagues; be aware of what you eat and how you exercise. The most liberated, healthy and happy individuals that I have met on my travels in the world are undoubtedly elderly members of a family who live with their children and who participate in the family and maintain a simple but orderly lifestyle. They are always up early. They chew their food very, very well. They are curious. They have no fear. Their family takes care of any financial concerns. They go to bed early. They eat simply. They keep active. There is a parallel here between developing health and developing wealth. Individuals who appear healthy will undoubtedly have a natural self-control, whether this is in how they eat, how they exercise or their attitude towards themselves. They are not necessarily fanatical but they are quietly disciplined about maintaining their health. Wealthy people are much the same. They are not lazy about money, they do not just expect it to arrive, they are working on it, cultivating it and undoubtedly very disciplined in the way they use it. How many times have you shared a bill with a wealthy person and they have divided it accurately down to the last cent or penny! It is just their natural discipline.

The real gift that oriental healing can provide us with is understanding the importance of preventing problems. This shows up, in Feng Shui, as the importance in deciding where to build a home, the immediate landscape, appreciating the influence of the surrounding buildings, careful planning of the interior for the ultimate benefit of the occupants. This is preventive medicine. In the healing arts, most of the emphasis is on the prevention of disease – advising individuals about their diet, their exercise, their breathing and how to maintain strong Chi. On the other hand, the emphasis from the Western point of view is more about curing and fixing things, whether this is bringing so-called 'cures' into a home or office to re-balance the Chi or using surgery or biomedical treatments to 'cure' a problem of health.

True freedom is the capacity to be responsible for your health and the direction your life takes. Being responsible translates into 'the ability to respond', and that ability is undoubtedly based on our intuition. We all have the choice to decide what we wish to do with our lives rather than having it dictated to us by other circumstances, other people or the limitations of our health. The choice is ours. I wish you an exciting journey that continues well beyond this ten-day programme.

FOOD GLOSSARY

---

amasake	a sweet custard made from cultured rice or other grain
aduki	a small red bean
bancha	the twigs and stems from Japanese tea bush, also known as kukicha
barley malt or malt extract	a natural sweetener made from sprouted barley
bonito flakes	dried, flaked tuna
brown rice vinegar	a naturally brewed vinegar from brown rice
buckwheat	a hardy grain eaten in form of kasha or soba noodles
flame deflector	a round metal disc placed under pots or pressure cookers to distribute heat evenly and prevent burning
ginger	pungent root tuber used as a seasoning in cooking
gomashio	a condiment from roasted sesame seeds and sea salt (recipe p. 215)
kombu	dried kelp sea vegetable
kukicha	see bancha
kuzu	vegetable root powder from wild vine
millet	small yellow grain
miso	bean paste made with soybeans and salt and grains
mugi miso	miso made from soybeans, barley, salt and water, preferably unpasteurised and aged 18 months
sauerkraut	shredded cabbage and sea salt which is pressed and pickled
sea salt	salt produced from salt water
shoyu	traditionally, naturally made soy sauce. Made from soybeans, wheat, water and sea salt
soba	Japanese noodles containing buckwheat
tahini	a butter made from sesame seeds (a puree of ground sesame seeds)
tofu	soybean curd made from soybeans, rich in protein
udon	Japanese wheat noodles
wakame	green leafy sea vegetable, kelp

Note: most of these foods will be readily available in a wholefood store, but don't give up on your local healthfood or Japanese shop. All the ingredients are on the wholesale lists and a good shopkeeper will be glad to order them for you if asked.

RESOURCES

Chi Kung
Healing Tao Centre,
188 Old Street,
London EC1V 9BP
Tel: 0700 078 1195
e mail: healingtao@prynet.co.uk

Shiatsu
The Shiatsu Society,
The Interchange Studios,
Dalby Street,
London NW5 3NQ
Tel: 0171 813 7772
Fax: 0171 813 7773

Feng Shui
The Feng Shui Society,
P.O. Box 83
Camberley
Surrey GU15 1XE
Tel: 07050 289200

Tai Chi
The Tai Chi Union for Great Britain,
102 Felsham Road,
London SW15 1DQ
Tel: 0171 352 7716

Yoga
British Wheel of Yoga,
1 Hamilton Place,
Boston Road,
Sleaford,
Lincolnshire NG34 7ES
Tel: 01529 306 851

Aromatherapy
Aromatherapy Organisations Council,
3 Latymer Close,
Braybrooke,
Leicester LE16 8LN
Tel: 01858 434242

Macrobiotics
The Macrobiotic Association of Great Britain,
377 Edgware Road,
London W2 1BT
Tel: 07050 138419

Macrobiotic Foods – Mail Order
Pure,
8 Victory Place,
London SE19 3RW
Tel: 0181 771 4522

The '10-Day Re-balance Programme'
For further information regarding:
• workshops
• consultations
Contact: Jon Sandifer,
P.O. Box 69,
Teddington
Middlesex TW11 9SH
England
Tel/Fax 0181 977 8988
email: Jon – Sandifer @ Compuserve. Com